The
Martial Artist's
Book
of Yoga

The Martial Artist's Book of Yoga

Improve Flexibility,
Balance and Strength for
- Higher Kicks
- Faster Strikes
- Smoother Throws
- Safer Falls
- Stronger Stances

Lily Chou
with Kathe Rothacher

FOREWORD BY Dr. Norman G. Link, 6th dan

PHOTOGRAPHS BY Andy Mogg

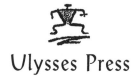

Ulysses Press

Published in the United States by
Ulysses Press
P.O. Box 3440
Berkeley, CA 94703
www.ulyssespress.com

Library of Congress Control Number 2005922408
ISBN 1-56975-472-1

Printed in Canada by Transcontinental Printing

10 9 8 7 6 5 4 3 2 1

Design	Robles-Aragón
Cover photography	Andy Mogg, except front top image © Gettyimages.com
Editorial and Production	Claire Chun, Tamara Kowalski, Matt Orendorff, Steven Zah Schwartz, Samantha Glorioso
Models	Jon Bertsch, Lily Chou, Adriana Espinosa, Percy Luu
Index	Sayre Van Young

Distributed by Publishers Group West

Please Note
This book has been written and published strictly for informational purposes,
and in no way should be used as a substitute for consultation with health care
professionals. You should not consider educational material herein to be the
practice of medicine or to replace consultation with a physician or other medical
practitioner. The author and publisher are providing you with information in this
work so that you can have the knowledge and can choose, at your own risk, to act
on that knowledge. The author and publisher also urge all readers to be aware
of their health status and to consult health care professionals before beginning
any health program, including changes in dietary habits.

Table of Contents

Foreword

If you are reading these words then you are one of the rare few that have chosen to do so. For that reason alone you deserve an explanation as to why the authors of this marvelous book have asked me to contribute a few words. My name will mean nothing to you; suffice it to say that I am a well-meaning person who has spent four decades practicing various martial arts, the last 28 years of them at the University of California at Berkeley. While I have abused, misused, and suffused my body with the rigors that the martial arts require (thus incurring the requisite number of injuries), I would not trade that time and experience for anything. HOWEVER, had this book been available to me when I started all those decades ago (and had I had the wisdom to pick it up and read it), I am convinced that today I would be all the better for it.

The Martial Artist's Book of Yoga is a long overdue project that helps return the martial arts to the world of a normal adult. Since the late 1960s, the martial arts have been associated with young, hyper, mostly male athletes who, for various reasons, wreak violence upon the world. The "art" in the term "martial art" has been lost, and with it the centuries-old attraction of martial exercise for all people, from the very young to the very old. Most traditional martial arts emphasized the essential interrelationship between mind and body. Unfortunately, the healthy philosophical as well as psychological aspects of the martial arts have eroded with the rush of competitions, from local events to the Olympics. This book not only can help all levels of martial arts practitioners but in a new way guides one in the direction of reintroducing both the physical and mental aspects of physical training.

I encourage everyone to find a nice quiet corner someplace and join me in enjoying and benefitting from this great book on human origami.

Dr. Norman G. Link, 6th *dan* yongmudo
Associate Director, Martial Arts Program
University of California at Berkeley

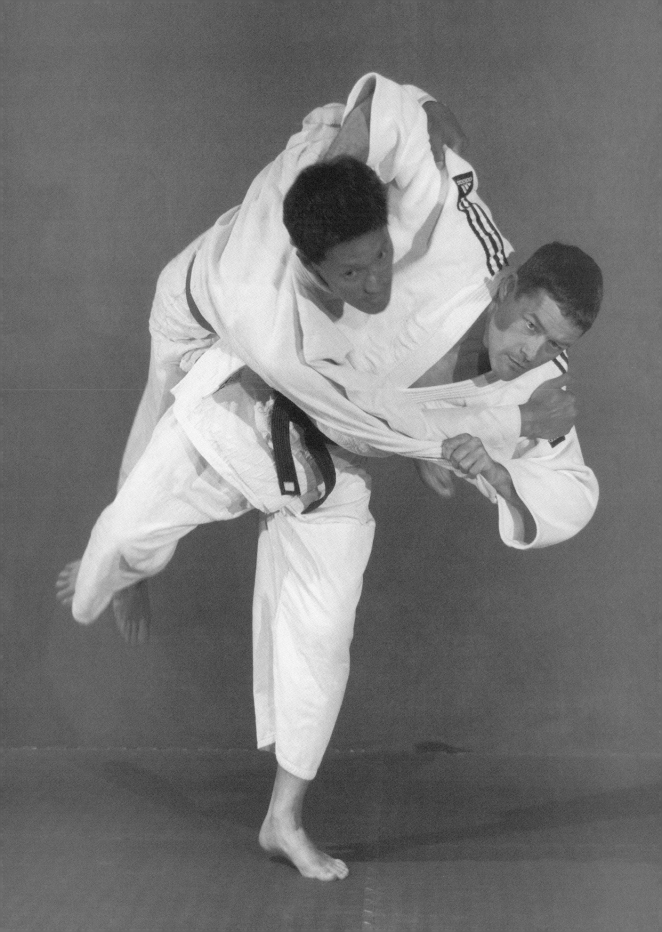

Preface

Welcome to *The Martial Artist's Book of Yoga*, a guide to improving your martial arts skills with the ancient practice of yoga. While the martial arts and yoga might seem like natural partners, even people who practice both don't always consider how deeply complementary they are. This book explores in detail the specific, practical ways yoga can benefit all forms of martial arts training, from honing particular techniques to enhancing your overall conditioning and awareness.

Count me among the people who took a long time to recognize the positive impact yoga could have on my martial arts training. Initially when I tried yoga, it wasn't specifically to improve

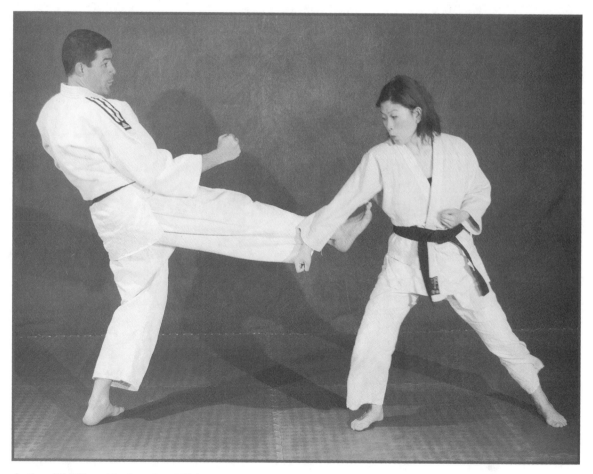

Author Lily Chou blocks a front kick.

my martial arts practice, but to undo injuries. The thought that I could become a better martial artist by practicing something presumably unrelated—yoga—had never occurred to me. But having trained in the Korean martial art of hapkido for six years and in taekwondo, another Korean discipline, for three, I had acquired an alarming number of neoprene supports and braces to hold my body together. These braces basically kept my various armored joints from reaching their pain zones, but they restricted movement and inhibited strengthening. Surely there was some way to correct the self-damage I had unwittingly done over the years and restore the flexibility and range of motion I had once enjoyed. Yoga, known for its therapeutic properties, seemed a logical thing to try.

Despite this motivation, I was bored to tears with my first yoga class. I remember standing in what the instructor called "Warrior I," holding the pose beyond the point where my quads were burning and my arms shaking. But my mind, accustomed to obvious outward goals such as striking a target or rolling forward in a straight line, didn't know what to do with itself. I'm sure it probably emitted a long silent shriek until we were allowed to move into a different pose. Yoga was so quiet and . . . introverted. My body was willing but my mind was not ready.

It would be another year before I attempted yoga again (for the same reason). This time, perhaps because of Kathe Rothacher's refreshing teaching style, I began noticing the similarities between yoga and the martial arts. But it wasn't until the following year, when I started teaching hapkido and deconstructing its various techniques, that I was convinced that yoga is indeed a great complement to martial arts training. It's no coincidence that some yoga poses resemble techniques in your martial arts repertoire. The two are not disparate entities—martial arts may even originate from yoga, as you'll read in the What Is Yoga section.

Whatever the relationship between yoga and the martial arts, with this book I hope you, too, gain improvements in both your martial arts training and life.

Lily Chou
September 2005

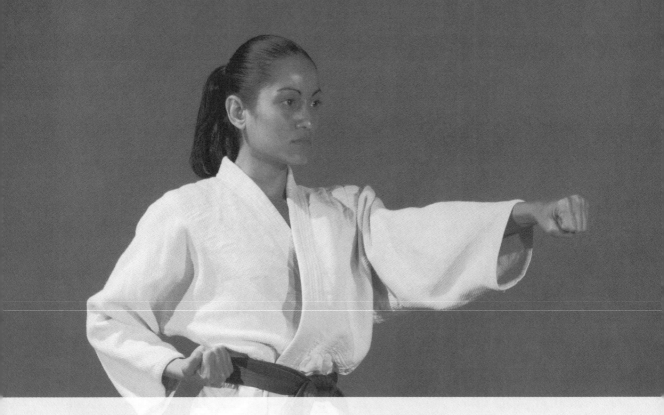

Part 1

Overview

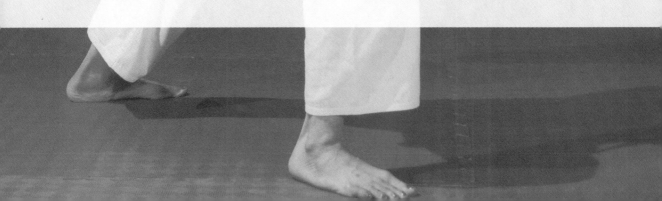

What Is Yoga

For all its current popularity, the age-old Indian practice of yoga still retains an elusive past. It may have existed as far back as 3000 B.C.E.—excavations in the Indus Valley have yielded stone seals depicting figures performing yoga *asanas* (or poses). These discoveries have led scholars to surmise that yoga evolved from shamanistic practices that flourished in that ancient civilization. But while we lack a definitive understanding of its origins, yoga's continuing vitality as a philosophy, art, and science is clear.

The word "yoga" basically means "union." It comes from the Sanskrit root *yuj*, which translates as "to yoke" or "to bind," referring to the ultimate ideal of yoga as a way to completely integrate mind, body, and spirit. Over hundreds of years many methods and specialties of practice have developed, ranging from intense physical exercises to esoteric meditations such as absorption in total silence. In the second century B.C.E., in an effort to standardize the multitude of yoga forms that had arisen, an Indian sage named Patanjali composed the Yoga Sutras. There he outlined the eight aspects of yoga:

1. *yama* (self-restraint); 2. *niyama* (observance of purity, devotion, and study); 3. *asana* (physical exercises); 4. *pranayama* (breath control); 5. *pratyahara* (withdrawal from the senses); 6. *dharana* (concentration); 7. *dhyana* (meditation); and 8. *samadhi* ("enlightenment").

Although some Western practitioners may actively engage in aspects of yoga such as breath control and meditation, the vast majority don't venture beyond the physical poses. The martial arts, however, more or less demand developing self-restraint, devotion, breath control, and concentration, among other things, when martial artists endeavor to improve the form, execution, and understanding of their techniques.

Legend persists that the martial arts as we know them derive from Prince Bodhidharma's visit to the Shaolin Temple in China in the sixth century B.C.E. Bodhidharma (who eventually founded the Zen branch of Buddhism—*zen* is derived from the Chinese word *ch'an*, which in turn comes from the Sanskrit *dhyana*), advocated meditation as the key to attaining enlightenment. The Shaolin monks, however, were so out of shape that their minds were unable to focus on the task at hand. So, perhaps borrowing from yogic systems where physical postures prepare the body for long periods of meditation, Bodhidharma developed a number of exercises (including the Eighteen Hands of the Lo Han) for the monks to train in. This exercise is claimed to have evolved into Shaolin Kung Fu.

Other conjectures about the origins of martial arts and yoga involve the many animal forms and other techniques that emulate natural processes. Whatever the historical or legendary sources, they all point to the same ultimate root: people with highly developed awareness of natural forms and processes showed how these relate to human movement—and, in turn, how to develop that very awareness.

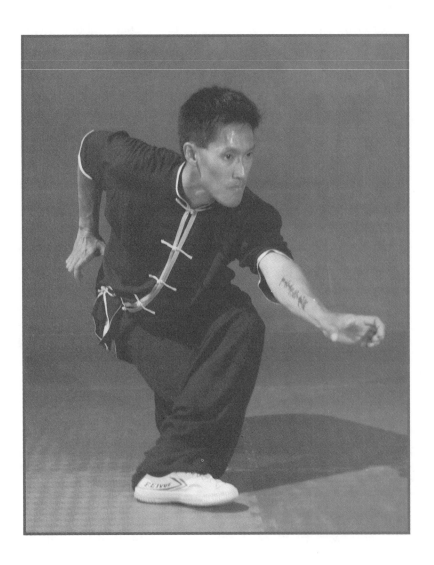

The Martial Artist's Book of Yoga

Benefits of Yoga for Martial Artists

The millennia-old Indian tradition of Hatha yoga (a style of yoga that emphasizes three of yoga's eight aspects: physical poses, breath control, and meditation) is well-known for its therapeutic properties, and millions of people around the world reap countless daily benefits (such as improving digestion, reducing stress, and relieving arthritis) from their practice. The most commonly held belief about *asanas*, or poses, is that they are simply fancy forms of stretches, useful only to those people who seek to increase their flexibility. But try yoga just once and you'll quickly learn that yoga contributes to your body's function in other, far-reaching ways.

Regardless of whether you've had previous yoga experience, and regardless of whether you're a beginning karate student who's having trouble chambering your sidekicks or a veteran judoka who can't remember the last time you had full range of motion in your knees, the poses in this book will transform you from the inside out, translating into better ability to perform the martial arts techniques that challenge you. After a few yoga sessions, you'll start noticing your body's weaknesses and habits that affect your martial arts performance as well as your day-to-day being: hunching over your computer, slouching while in line at the checkout stand. Luckily, this awareness is the first step to overcoming your unhealthy movement patterns.

Of course, this is not to say yoga will improve your martial arts if you stop practicing martial arts—it won't. Your martial arts techniques will only improve if you practice those techniques. But like the martial arts, yoga develops a disciplined mind, body, and spirit, and enhances the connection between all three. It serves as an avenue through which you can observe your body's weaknesses and strengths and correct those imbalances, allowing movement to come more freely and easily. The following elements have a significant impact on all martial arts training.

Flexibility

Flexibility is the range of motion of a specific joint. A surprising number of people place flexibility low on the fitness scale, but flexibility isn't just for doing split kicks and evading armbars in grappling situations—it's the key to moving properly and preventing injury. Good flexibility allows your body to get into position more quickly and with less effort, and reduces the risk of getting hurt.

Although the physical structure of a particular joint can limit your range of motion (and flexibility in one place doesn't necessarily apply to another—being able to touch your nose with your toes doesn't mean you'll be able to reach your hand down your back), you can permanently improve your range through regular stretching and muscular balance. Think of the various yoga poses as super-stretches: while "regular" stretches target specific muscles or body parts, *asanas* can simultaneously stretch several muscles, at the same time building balance, strength, body control, and a host of other things. Most *asanas* also promote a supple spine and flexible hips, which are vital for fluidity, speed, and power in all martial arts techniques, regardless of style practiced. And yoga routines—sequences of *asanas*—can truly improve flexibility everywhere.

Strength

Strength is the ability of all your muscles to perform work via their intended movements. Although the martial arts train both sides of the body, you'll notice that one side is generally weaker than the other and never seems to catch up to the stronger side, no matter how much you may practice. The chronic overuse of certain muscles is common in all physical activities, and this creates muscular imbalances that can pull joints out of alignment—ultimately resulting

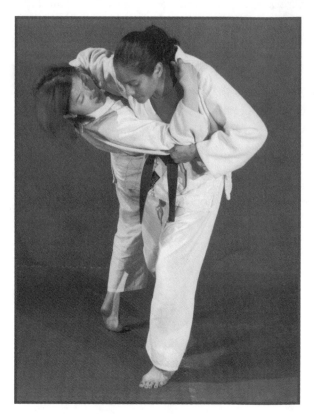

in painful movement and a higher likelihood of injury.

An *asana* triggers the appropriate muscles for a particular movement and works them equally, especially when you hold the pose for an extended period of time. Weak muscles are allowed to develop and overused ones are given the opportunity to rest. The *asanas* also train the body to function as a unit—an obvious benefit, considering not one martial arts technique is achieved solely by the use of a single isolated muscle. Even something like a basic front punch, ostensibly an upper body movement, requires a shift of the hips to generate power from the legs. Muscles strengthened through the balanced and complementary approach of yoga conserve energy, make work easier, and reduce the risk of injury.

Alignment

Proper body alignment, which includes good posture, benefits every aspect of how you move, from walking to picking up the phone, to rolling, to pulling your jujitsu partner off-balance. If your body is misaligned even slightly, you must work harder to perform an action. Not only does use of inappropriate muscles reduce your body's response time—consistent misuse will eventually create more imbalance in your body, and likely reduce your range of motion and increase pain. Proper alignment results in a stronger body, and is crucial for economy of movement, speed, a good center of gravity, and reduced risk of injury.

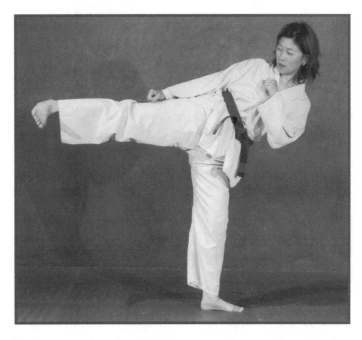

Balance

Balance is something the body continuously attempts to achieve. It's what allows you to sit, stand, walk, reach up and change a lightbulb. The information the brain receives from the body regarding its position in time and space affects balance, as does the alignment of the joints in the body. Many martial arts techniques require you to balance in specialized positions. Spin hook kicks, for instance, involve rotating on one foot as the other leg whips out; forward body drops have you balancing on the balls of your feet as you load on your partner and then flip them over. Balance lets you execute such techniques and also guarantees faster recovery post-execution. Harmonizing with the natural flow of energy, as practiced in styles such as in jujitsu, aikido, and judo, leads to a dynamic balance that's critical in protecting the knees, hips, and back from injury.

Body Awareness/Control

Before you can get your body to do what you want it to do, you must be aware of how accurately your body responds to your commands. Does the reality of what it's doing match your perception of what you're attempting to do? For instance, when you're in a good front stance (or Warrior I), are your hips square, as they should be? Or do you only think they are? Unfortunately, martial arts techniques are usually done at a speed that does not allow much biofeedback and introspection.

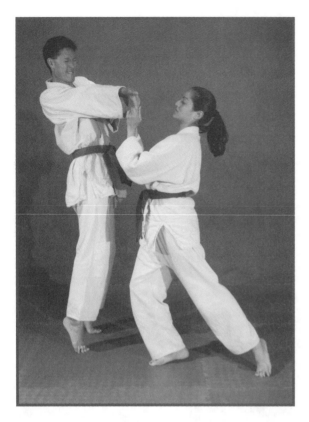

Getting into *asanas* heightens body awareness and alignment, magnifying the connection between your mind and your muscles. Holding the positions forces you to feel which muscles are struggling to hold you in place and which ones don't need to be involved. Once you're aware of what your body is doing, you can begin to control its voluntary and involuntary actions. You'll start noticing more frequently if your limbs are flailing during a grappling session, and you'll pull them close to your body before your opponent can catch them in a lock. You're likely to gain power and speed in your strikes and kicks when you no longer waste effort in unnecessary countermotion (like torquing your shoulders to better propel a kick) or early "telegraph" of your movements (detrimental in a competitive or sparring situation). More complete control of your body and its functions also heightens your ability to judge distance, whether striking a target or evading an opponent; conserve energy by refraining from unnecessary movement; and focus the appropriate amount of power for the desired degree of impact.

Breath Control

Everyone breathes, true, but proper breathing takes practice. The slow, mindful breathing of yoga, as opposed to the rapid, shallow breaths that come when anxious or rushed, results in improved endurance, balance, stamina, and power; reduced recovery time; relaxed muscles; and a calm mind. It also fosters efficient delivery of oxygen to muscles. In addition (paradoxically, it might seem), yogic breathing sharpens your vision and enhances your ability to move quickly and fluidly.

Just as you synchronize your exhale, or *kihap/kiai* (Korean/Japanese for "spirit yell"), with your strike, kick, or fall, you exhale when applying exertion in a yoga pose. Exhaling explosively in conjunction with martial arts techniques helps increase power or safeguard against injury; breathing while in a yoga pose works to unify the mind and body with the breath and to clear any blocks that restrict the flow of *prana* (or *chi*, in Chinese; *ki* in Japanese). Most advanced martial artists learn to channel this vital internal energy to augment their physical strength.

Focus

Keeping a clear, calm mind in the face of adversity is perhaps the hardest thing to cultivate, martial artist or not. The calmer you are, the more clearly you can assess a situation and respond appropriately. Slowing down internally allows you to hear and see more, as well as make better choices for action. The mindfulness required of, and enhanced in, each yoga pose develops focus.

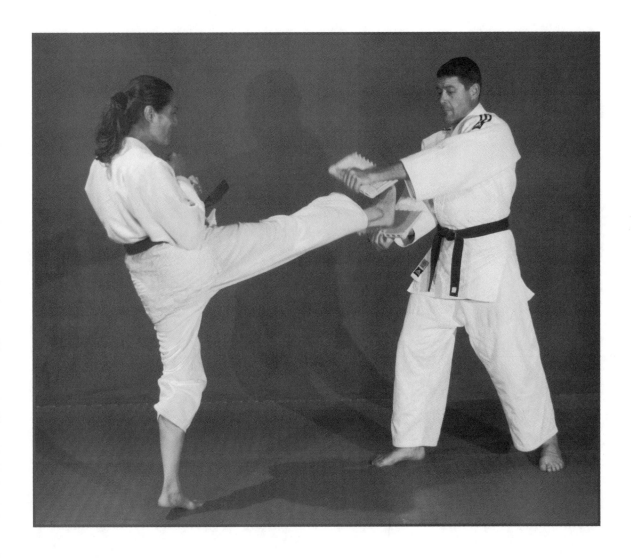

Part 2
Getting Started

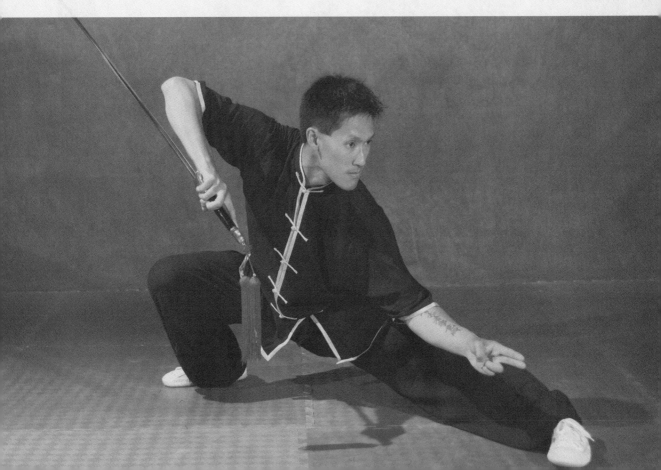

Martial Artist's Yoga

With hundreds of martial arts styles practiced today, martial arts techniques number in the thousands, and even the same technique will vary from style to style and from school to school. Despite this diversity, these techniques share similar underlying foundations. *The Martial Artist's Book of Yoga* breaks down the techniques into six general groups: falls/rolls, grappling moves, joint locks (which, unlike grappling, include those done from standing), kicks, hand strikes/blocks, and throws. Each section provides an overview of the family of techniques and identifies the physical elements required to perform them. The book then describes how yoga can complement training in that area and recommends several *asanas* chosen specifically to benefit that genre of techniques.

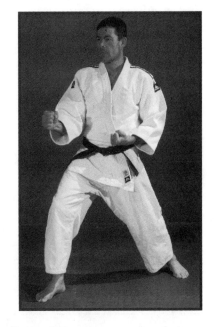

You need not feel intimidated by the material in this book. We include only "practical" postures that may be challenging but, for the most part, not impossible to perform. In addition, please note that the models featured here are *not* yoga professionals—we are all martial artists with varying degrees of yoga experience. Some of us may have tight hips or shoulders, others may have over-conditioned quads or poor balance. Regardless of our personal physiological quirks, we all attempted the poses to the best of our abilities, as should you. Improvement of ourselves and our bodies can only be achieved through trying.

Since most poses can be done several ways, we've provided instruction that best supports martial arts function and form. For instance, Warrior I and Powerful are commonly practiced with the arms extended overhead and hands held shoulder-width apart; this book has you clasp your hands together to increase the stretch in your shoulders. In addition, this book presents modifications and variations to either simplify or intensify a pose. When applicable, some poses include a martial arts "challenge," which typically adds movement to a static pose.

Yoga Basics

Time & Place

Yoga can be done any time of the day, and anywhere there is space to extend your limbs and body. Some people prefer working in a quiet place; others find no problem tuning out the distractions of busier locales. Beginners may find quiet spaces more productive, but practice wherever you're most comfortable. Depending on the intensity and duration of the practice and the poses performed, your yoga experience may be stimulating, calming, energizing, or relaxing. Your practice can be as short or long as you'd like, but the most benefit seems to come from a session that lasts at least 15 minutes. Perform these poses prior to your martial arts training as a way to prepare the body for further activity, and/or after training as a way to release, rebalance, and relax your muscles and calm your mind. You can also practice yoga on non-martial arts days for increased conditioning.

Clothing & Equipment

Wear comfortable clothing that does not restrict your movement. It's best to practice yoga with bare feet for better contact with the floor. Equipment is not necessary, but you may find it help-

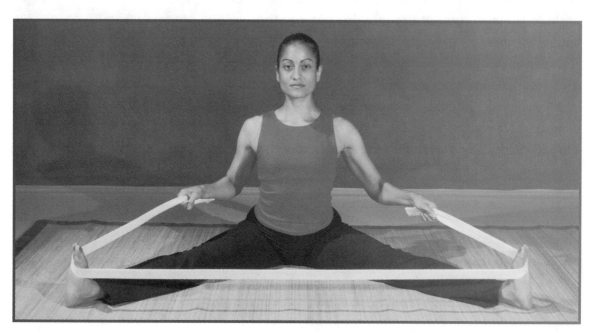

The Martial Artist's Book of Yoga

ful. Sticky mats can prevent you from slipping on carpet or other surfaces. Blocks can help promote stability, alignment, and balance. Straps may enhance flexibility.

The Practice

A typical yoga session begins with meditation, proceeds into a warm-up, moves on to poses, and then ends with rest.

MEDITATION   This clears the mind and prepares mind, body, and spirit for a mindful workout. You can do this either standing or sitting comfortably. However you choose to meditate, focus on your breath and its interaction with your body, and try to clear your mind of the events/anxieties of your day.

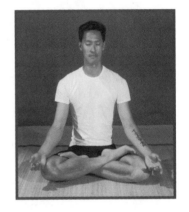

WARM-UP   Just as you wouldn't leap into flying back kicks without first warming up, perhaps by doing some stretch kicks then throwing a few standing back kicks, you shouldn't bend and twist into Reverse Triangle without preparing your body beforehand. The most basic yoga warm-up is the Sun Salutation (see page 32). This series of movements lengthens, strengthens, stretches, and extends most of your major muscles in preparation for other *asanas*. Of course, you can always raise your heart rate and warm your muscles with a few dozen jumping jacks or several minutes of running in place, but these exercises don't prepare you physically and mentally as well as several Sun Salutations can.

POSES   There are several hundred *asanas* in practice today. This book presents 45 (or 46, counting Corpse Pose in the Rest section below) poses, which may range from being simple to completely impossible, depending on a host of things, including your physiology, energy level, and mood. Keep in mind that perfecting the pose is not the goal, although you will definitely improve with practice.

Breathing   Some instructors prefer that you inhale and exhale through your nose; others ask that you inhale through your nose and exhale through your mouth. For the course of your martial arts yoga practice, it doesn't matter which you do, as long as you remember to breathe and work on evening out both parts of your breath. Try not to hold your breath, especially when you're struggling with a pose. Breathing smoothly and regularly can only help you. Here are some basic yoga breathing rules:

1) Exhale when you fold your torso toward your legs (such as when you bend forward) or when you move a limb or limbs toward your torso (such as when you bring your knee to your chest).

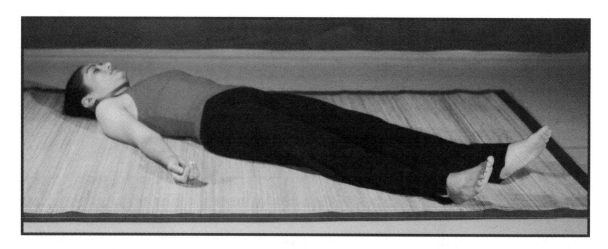

2) Inhale when you lift your torso away from your legs (such as when you move out of a forward bend) or when you move a limb or limbs away from your torso (such as when you raise your arms).

Transitioning   Some instructors teach poses without transition and/or any form of continuity; others flow from one pose to the next. We've organized the poses in each martial arts section in the best order that they should be performed, basically from standing to sitting to back-bending to inverting. Once you become familiar with several *asanas*, you can experiment with transitioning from one into another. For instance, try moving smoothly from Mountain into Warrior I into Warrior II into Triangle into Half Moon. Or Staff into Seated Forward Bend into Bound Angle into Bharadvaja's Pose. You'll find that your body will respond differently than if you were to do each pose singly. Transitioning in yoga is similar to combining various martial arts techniques in fluid fashion, whether you pair kicks with hand strikes, or move from a mount position in grappling into a scarf hold.

REST   Corpse Pose (or *Savasana*, pictured above) is often done after a session of yoga in order to relax your body and calm your mind. This allows your body to reflect and absorb all the benefits of your practice.

Start by lying on your back, either with your legs straight along the floor or knees bent and feet flat on the floor, whichever is more comfortable. Extend your arms out a bit from your sides. Close your eyes and resolve not to move or fidget. Breathe smoothly and evenly, focusing on your breath, letting go of any tension you become aware of. Allow every part of your body to sink into the floor and rest. After a few minutes, exhale and roll to one side. Take a few breaths, then push your hands against the floor, keeping your arms connected to your torso. With an exhale, bring your upper body to a sitting position.

Special Notes

Don't forgo the fundamentals

While it's okay to do all the poses in one section and stop there, for example, do not disregard the Fundamentals section. The poses here are "fundamental" because they serve as the basis for most other poses and also help improve the function of your body, no matter which martial arts you train in. If you practice judo, you'd want to check out the throws, falls/rolls, grappling, and joint locks sections; if you train in taekwondo, you'd want to look into kicks and strikes/blocks. Or you can jump around, doing what you feel your body needs. But remember, training comprehensively will help you the most, sometimes in unexpected ways—and whichever martial arts you identify with, you should always perform the Fundamental poses.

Slow down

The combative and/or defensive nature of martial arts techniques make its practitioners tend to execute movements quickly. Beginners often sacrifice their form and power in their haste to complete a maneuver, but this speed isn't always a deliberate choice—it's easier to perform techniques quickly, since

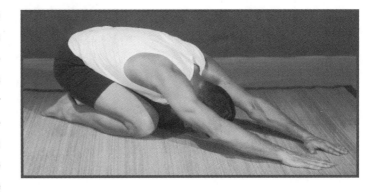

slow movements require considerably more control. To gain the most out of your yoga practice, strive to move in and out of poses mindfully. Don't hurry. Remember to breathe. Permit your body to reap the benefits of the pose by sensing your asymmetry, feeling your muscles adjusting, stretching, and strengthening in order to find the pose. This awareness will transfer directly into your martial arts performance.

Listen to your body

Shaking or quivering muscles are common when you first begin practicing yoga. No need for alarm—this signals that your muscles are working in a new way. With time, as your body gets stronger and adapts, the trembling will diminish. However, pay attention to whether you experience any pain when entering or holding a pose. You should know the difference between good and bad pain. Good pain isn't really "pain," but tightness or slight discomfort, such as when you bend over to put on your shoes the day after you've run five miles. This sensation should subside as you breathe into the pose and the muscles accommodate.

Bad pain is sharp and shooting and generally occurs in the knees, back, wrists, or other joints. If you encounter this variety as you enter a pose, back off immediately. Assess what you may have been doing, then mindfully try again—more slowly, with less pressure. If the same pain arises, stop and skip the pose. If you have pre-existing weaknesses—ankles, knees, lower back, or wrists, for instance—enter a questionable pose cautiously, ready to stop immediately if you feel bad pain. Do not attempt to push through this pain as you might when training in martial arts—it is not the purpose of these *asanas* to aggravate any painful conditions or, worse, cause one.

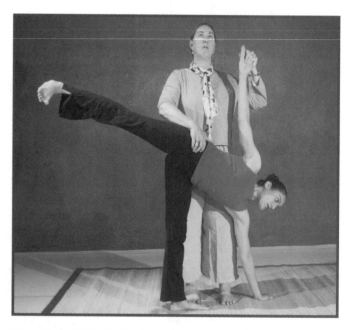

Check your alignment

Consider a punch: your forearm, wrist, and knuckles should lie on the same plane. Just a minor bend in the wrist not only weakens the power of the punch, it increases the chance of hurting your wrist. Alignment when performing yoga poses is similarly important: when you're properly

Co-author Kathe Rothacher makes some adjustments.

aligned, there's no break in energy flow and often the pose is easier to hold. Once you're in your pose, take a moment to check that your shoulders aren't hiked up around your ears, that your toes are pointing the right direction, that your leg is as straight as it can possibly be. If something's not quite right, breathe, notice, observe, and adjust yourself. Continue monitoring your body as you hold the pose.

Switch sides

Traditionally, when doing poses that don't use both the left and right sides of your body symmetrically (e.g., Warrior I, Triangle, Eagle), you begin with your right side, such that your left foot is

The Martial Artist's Book of Yoga

forward and your right leg is behind, or you bend to one side first. Consider occasionally switching the side that you start on so that your less powerful side (often the left side if you're right-handed) gets an opportunity to develop more fully. In addition to switching legs or twisting to the other side, don't forget to change the clasp of your hands when doing poses that require you to interlock your fingers.

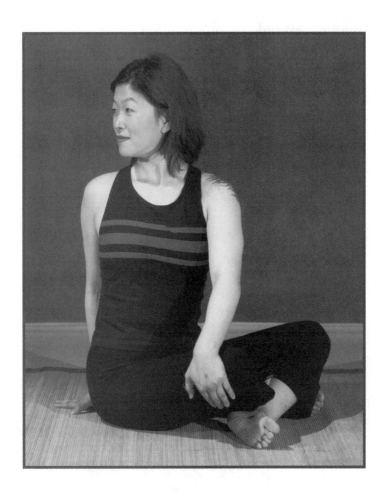

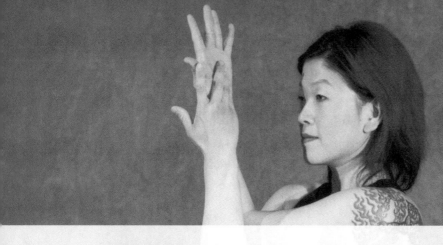

Part 3

The Poses

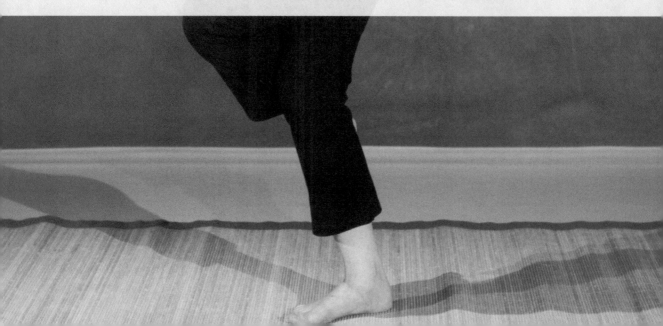

Fundamentals

These Fundamental poses serve as the foundations of many other poses in this book. They improve common martial arts stances and benefit martial artists because of their overall warming, lengthening, and strengthening properties.

Mountain (Tadasana)

■ *tada* = mountain ■ (tah-DAHS-anna) ■

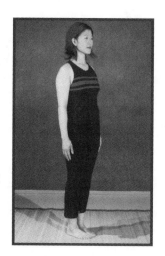

GENERAL BENEFITS: The foundation of all standing poses. This strengthens the legs, knees, and ankles; improves posture; teaches balance.

GETTING INTO POSE: Stand with your heels and the bases of your big toes touching, your weight evenly distributed between both feet. Lift your kneecaps toward your hips and tuck your pelvis slightly forward. Hang your arms along your sides and roll your shoulders back and down. Keep your head centered over your legs, and imagine that a string that runs from between your heels and through the center of your body is pulling the top of your head toward the ceiling.

Hold for 10 breaths.

Warrior I (Virabhadrasana I)

■ Virabhadra = a mighty warrior who was an incarnation of Shiva ■ (veer-ah-bah-DRAHS-anna) ■

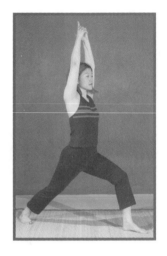

GENERAL BENEFITS: Similar to the front or bow stance, except the legs are narrower here. This strengthens the quads, knees, and ankles; stretches the hip flexors, legs, and shoulders; promotes proper hip alignment.

GETTING INTO POSE: From Mountain Pose, bring your arms overhead and clasp your hands, extending your index fingers to the ceiling. Step your right foot straight back and bend your left knee over your left ankle. Keeping your right leg straight and strong, turn your right foot out 45 degrees so that the heel is on the same line as your left foot. Gaze straight ahead.

Hold for 10 breaths. Repeat on the other side.

Warrior II (Virabhadrasana II)

■ Virabhadra = a mighty warrior who was an incarnation of Shiva ■ (veer-ah-bah-DRAHS-anna) ■

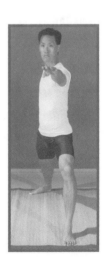

GENERAL BENEFITS: Strengthens the legs, knees, and ankles; stretches the legs, groin muscles, and shoulders; opens the hips and chest; promotes proper shoulder alignment

GETTING INTO POSE: From Mountain Pose, step your feet wide apart with your arms raised parallel to the floor, palms down. Keeping your hips facing forward, turn your right foot in 15 degrees and your left out 90 degrees. Bend your left knee so that it is in line with your ankle. With your head in line with your spine, turn your head to gaze out over your left hand.

Hold for 10 breaths. Repeat on the other side.

Side Angle (Parsvakonasana)

■ *parsva* = side; *kona* = angle ■ (parsh-vah-cone-AHS-anna) ■

GENERAL BENEFITS: Strengthens the legs, knees, and ankles; stretches the legs and sides of the torso; opens the hips

GETTING INTO POSE: From Mountain Pose, step your feet wide apart with your arms raised parallel to the floor, palms down. Keeping your hips facing forward, turn your right foot in 15 degrees and your left out 90 degrees. Bend your left knee so that it is in line with your ankle. Lean over your left thigh and place your hand next to the inside of your foot; extend your right hand toward the ceiling so that your arms create a line perpendicular to the floor. Turn your head to gaze at your top hand.

Hold for 10 breaths. Repeat on the other side.

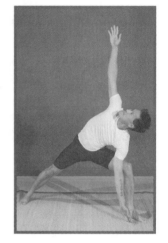

Intense Stretch (Uttanasana)

■ *ut* = intense; *tan* = to stretch ■ (OOT-tan-AHS-anna) ■

Also known as **Standing Forward Bend Pose**

GENERAL BENEFITS: Stretches the hamstrings, calves, and hips; strengthens the quads and knees

GETTING INTO POSE: From Mountain Pose, inhale and raise your arms overhead. Exhale and fold from your hips, lifting your kneecaps toward your hips, keeping your weight even on both feet. Place your hands on either side of your feet, fingers in line with your toes, and release your head toward the floor.

Hold for 10 breaths.

MODIFICATION: If you cannot touch the floor, hold an elbow in each hand or place your hands on your shins.

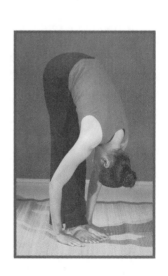

Downward-Facing Dog
(Adho Mukha Svanasana)

■ *adho* = downward; *mukha* = face; *svana* = dog ■
(AH-doh MOO-kah shvah-NAHS-anna) ■

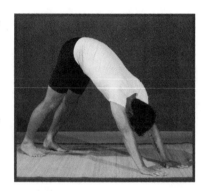

GENERAL BENEFITS: An all-over body stretch that may eventually become a resting pose. This strengthens the arms and legs; stretches the shoulders, hands, hamstrings, calves, and back.

GETTING INTO POSE: Kneel with your knees beneath your hips and hands, fingers spread wide apart and palms flat on the floor, beneath your shoulders. Tuck your toes under, push into your hands, and lift your hips to the ceiling. Lengthen your legs, reaching your heels toward the floor and your tailbone to the ceiling. Keep your head between your biceps.

Hold for 10 breaths.

Upward-Facing Dog
(Urdhva Mukha Svanasana)

■ *urdhva* = upward; *mukha* = face; *svana* = dog ■
(ERD-vah MOO-kah shvah-NAHS-anna) ■

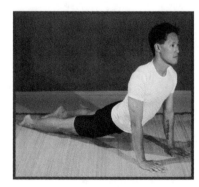

GENERAL BENEFITS: Stretches the chest, shoulders, and abs; strengthens the spine, arms, wrists, and butt

GETTING INTO POSE: Lie face down with your legs extended along the floor. Keeping your elbows by your sides, place your hands, fingers spread wide apart, on the floor by your waist so your forearms are perpendicular to the floor. Inhale as you straighten your arms to lift your head and chest, and press into the tops of your feet to raise your thighs off the floor. Roll your shoulders down and back.

Hold for 10 breaths.

The Martial Artist's Book of Yoga

Child's (Balasana)

■ *bala* = child ■ (bah-LAHS-anna) ■

GENERAL BENEFITS: A gentle resting pose that stretches the hips, quads, and ankles; releases the back and neck.

GETTING INTO POSE: Sit on your heels with the tops of your feet on the floor and your arms along your sides. Fold your torso forward onto your thighs as you extend your arms in front of you. Rest your forehead on the floor. Breathe into your ribs and feel them press into your thighs as they expand.

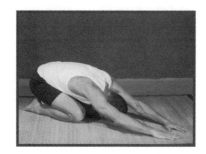

Hold for 10 breaths.

Staff (Dandasana)

■ *danda* = staff ■ (don-DAHS-anna) ■

GENERAL BENEFITS: The basis for many sitting poses. This strengthens the legs; stretches the arms and legs; opens the chest; promotes proper posture.

GETTING INTO POSE: Sit with your legs together and extended straight out in front of you. Imagine a string that runs from between your hips and through the center of your body pulling the top of your head to the ceiling. Press your palms into the floor just slightly behind each side of your hips, and roll your shoulders back and down.

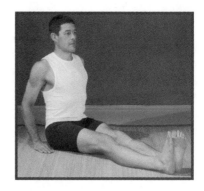

Hold for 10 breaths.

Sun Salutation

The Sun Salutation is a series of movements and *asanas* strung together to lengthen, strengthen, stretch, and extend most of your major muscles. It can be performed to warm up the body before moving on to more challenging poses, or simply as a complete practice in itself. The Sun Salutation has many permutations. The sequence shown uses all the Fundamental poses in this section.

1. Start in Mountain (page 27).

2. Inhale and arc your arms out to the sides and up above your head.

3. Exhale and, sweeping your arms out to the sides, fold at the hips into Intense Stretch (page 29). Place your hands or fingertips on the floor or your shins.

4. Inhale and arc your heart forward.

5. Exhale back into Intense Stretch Pose.

6. Press your hands firmly into the floor on either side of your feet. Keeping your arms strong, inhale and step both feet straight back into a push-up position (or Plank Pose).

7. Exhale and push your hips back into Downward-Facing Dog (page 30). Inhale.

8. Exhale and step your right foot, then your left, forward into Intense Stretch.

9. Inhale and slowly roll up your spine one vertebra at a time to bring yourself to Mountain Pose.

10. Exhale and step into Warrior I (page 28) with your left knee bent forward. Inhale.

11. Exhale into Warrior II (page 28) by reaching your left arm forward and right arm back. Inhale.

12. Exhale into Side Angle (page 29) by piercing your left arm forward, placing your left hand on the floor beside your foot, and reaching your right arm to the ceiling. Inhale.

13. Exhale back into Warrior II. Inhale.

14. Exhale into Warrior I. Inhale.

15. Exhale and reach both arms forward to place your hands on either side of your left foot. Step your left foot back into Plank. Inhale.

16. Exhale and lower down into Four-Limbed Staff (page 114).

17. Inhale as you push your chest through your arms into Upward-Facing Dog (page 30).

18. Exhale and push your hips back into Downward-Facing Dog. Inhale.

19. Exhale and step your left foot, then your right, forward into Intense Stretch Pose.

20. Inhale and slowly roll up your spine one vertebra at a time into Mountain Pose.

Once you are done with the sequence, repeat again, substituting "left" for "right" and "right" for "left" where appropriate. As a warm-up, do at least one full set. For those days when you don't have time to do other poses, perform at least three full Sun Salutations. Gradually try to flow from one step to another, synchronizing your breath with your movements as you do so.

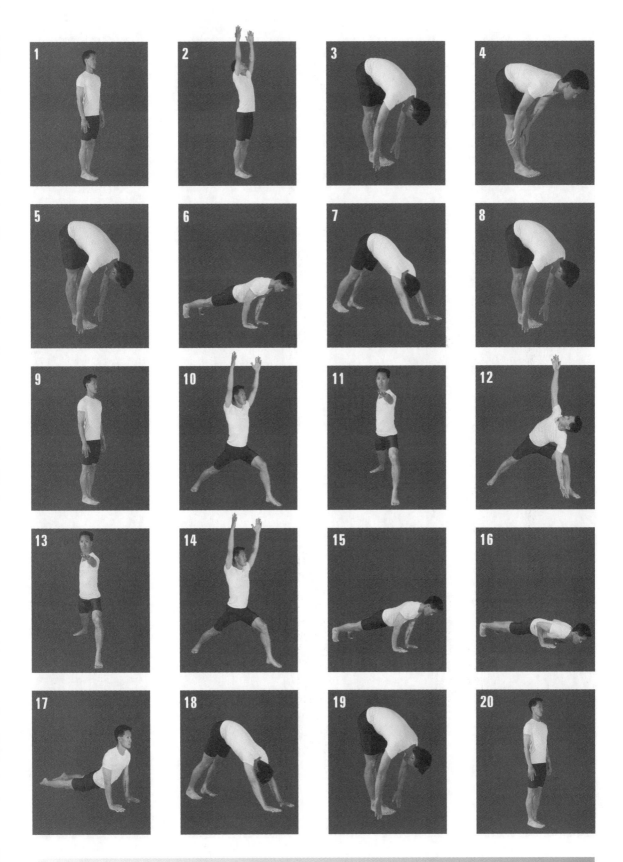

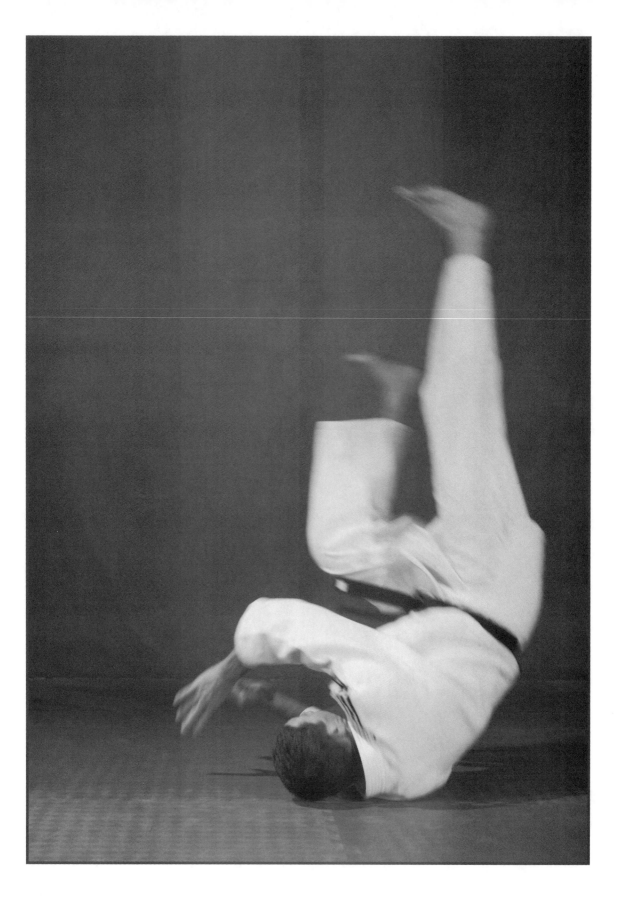

Falls/Rolls

One of the first things you learn in jujitsu, judo, aikido, or any other martial art that involves throws is how to fall. This group of techniques is called breakfalls, which can be jarring to the system and often leaves beginners' arms and legs red and tender. Rolls take longer to learn but, once mastered, offer softer, more fluid forms of protection. Rolls and falling techniques exist for a variety of situations and, when properly executed, they all serve to disperse the impact of hitting the ground and protect your most vital parts: head, neck, and spine.

KEY ANATOMY

All falls and rolls use the shoulders, back, legs, feet, and, for the most part, arms and hands. The abdominal muscles work to support the back.

Essential Elements

BODY AWARENESS/ALIGNMENT/CONTROL It takes a lot of practice before the many technical aspects of rolling and falling become second-nature. When rolling, you must simultaneously know where to put your hands, how to turn your head, when to push off, how to round your back, and how to tuck your legs so you get up with ease—all the while making sure every part of your body is properly aligned to protect your body. Falling has similar elements to take into consideration. Knowing where your body is at all times, and what it's doing, is the first step to gaining control of rolls and falls and preventing injury (such as clashing your ankles as you land or banging your elbows when you slap out at 90 degrees instead of the safer 45). Once you become aware of what your body's doing, you can begin to control all the elements to perform safer falls and rolls: using your legs to adjust the velocity and extent of your roll or fall so you don't hit your head or crunch your neck; tucking your chin and legs at the appropriate moment; rounding your back; slapping with your hands.

FLEXIBILITY A strong, supple spine is beneficial for all kinds of movement, and is particularly important when rolling and falling. Not only is a flexible spine more

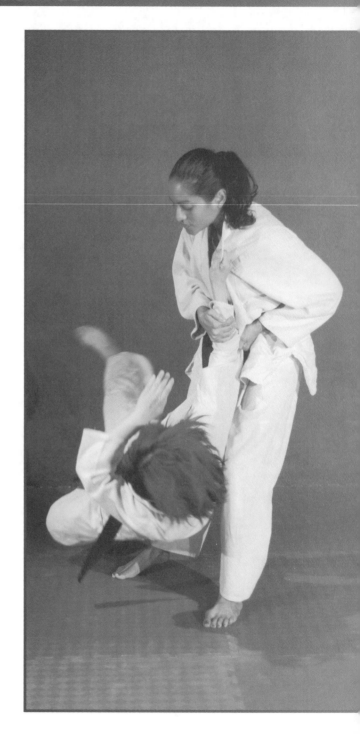

resilient to the constant impact it receives, its flexibility allows you to perform techniques better. Rolls become smoother when you're able to round your back (the difference between spinning a perfect wheel and one with a dent in it) and most falls feel softer when your back isn't rigid. Flexibility of the spine, shoulders, and hamstrings helps reduce the instances and degree of strain or injury to your back and upper body.

BALANCE   The need to roll or fall occurs when you're physically unbalanced, whether someone throws or strikes you, you fall off a bike, or you trip over your own feet. Knowing where your center of mass is helps you rotate properly and/or distribute your weight evenly as you fall, so no single part of your body receives the brunt of the impact. It also helps you recover your balance more quickly, letting you come to a stand or suitable defensive position, ready to perform a follow-up technique.

BREATH CONTROL   Just as you must use your arms to control the degree and rate of a fall or roll, you must *kihap/kiai* (Korean/Japanese for "spirit yell") as you hit the ground to maintain control of your

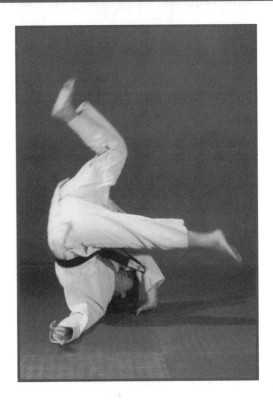

breath. Certainly breath control is important in the execution of all martial arts techniques. However, unlike forgetting to *kihap* when striking or kicking, which generally only leads to less powerful techniques, forgetting to deliberately force the air out of your lungs when you fall can result in getting it knocked out of you, leaving you winded and often incapacitated for several crucial seconds.

Benefits of Yoga

The Fundamental poses increase spine and hip mobility and improve alignment. Beyond that, all the poses in this section warm up and release the spine and the muscles often used in rolls and falls. They also restore muscular balance in your back and abs, preventing injury from overuse and misuse. Some of the poses also challenge your balance, promoting body awareness and control, while others strengthen your back, abs, and arms to better tolerate and disperse impact. All yoga poses, with their attention to breathing and body position, enhance breath control.

Poses for Falls/Rolls

Gate (*Parighasana*)

Boat (*Navasana*)

Bharadvaja's Pose I (*Bharadvajasana I*)

Locust (*Salabhasana*)

Camel (*Ustrasana*)

Plow (*Halasana*)

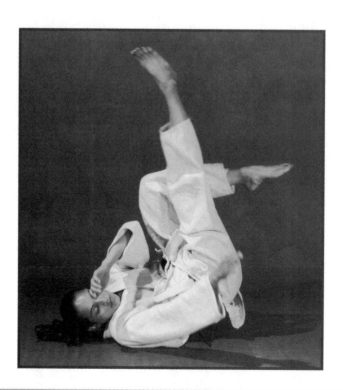

The Martial Artist's Book of Yoga

Other Poses

These poses that appear elsewhere in the book also benefit falls and rolls:

Intense Leg Extension III *(page 80):* stretches the hamstrings and shoulders

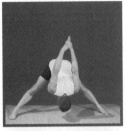

All-Limb *(page 70):* stretches the spine and shoulders; improves balance

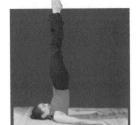

Four-Limbed Staff *(page 114):* strengthens the arms for slapping and supporting weight

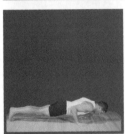

Vasishta's Pose *(page 116):* strengthens the arms for slapping and supporting weight; improves balance

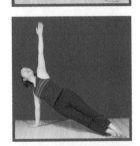

Half Lord of the Fishes *(page 62):* promotes hip and spine flexibility

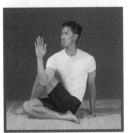

Sideways Extension *(page 96):* stretches the muscles used in forward rolls

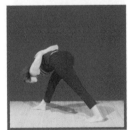

One-Legged King Pigeon *(page 104):* stretches the hips; warms up the muscles used in knee-under falls

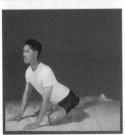

Cobra *(page 136):* reverses the compressing effect of rolls and falls

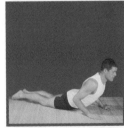

Seated Angle *(page 106):* releases the hamstrings and back

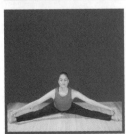

Crane *(page 120):* strengthens the arms for supporting weight; improves balance

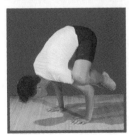

Gate (Parighasana)

■ *parigha* = bar used to latch a gate shut ■ (par-ee-GAHS-anna) ■

GENERAL BENEFITS: Stretches the sides of the torso and hips; strengthens the legs

VARIATION: Turn your raised palm down and gaze up at your biceps.

Martial arts application

BENEFITS: Reverses the compressing effect of rolls and side falls

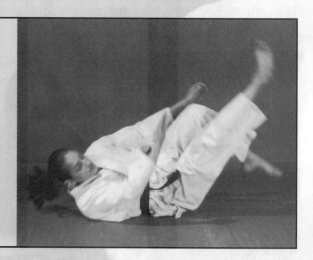

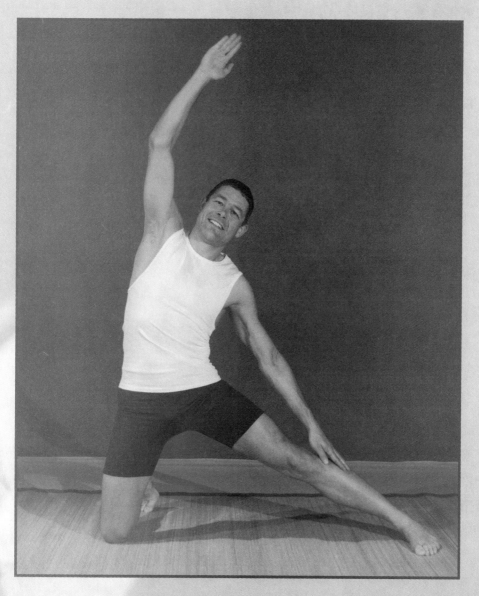

GETTING INTO POSE: Kneel with your knees and feet together and your hands on your hips. Inhale as you raise both arms to shoulder height and extend your left leg out to the side, sole on the floor and toes pointing forward. Exhale and slide your left hand to your left foot as your right arm arcs up over your head and reaches for your left foot. Keep your arms, head, torso, hips, and extended leg in one plane. Gaze straight ahead, keeping your head aligned with your spine.

Hold for 10 breaths. Repeat on the other side.

Boat (Navasana)

■ *nava* = boat ■ (nah-VAHS-anna) ■

GENERAL BENEFITS: Strengthens the abs, quads, hip flexors, and back

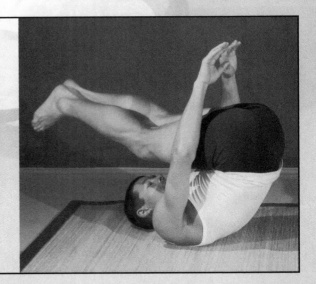

Martial arts application

BENEFITS: Improves ability to control the rotational rate of a roll/fall

CHALLENGE: Keeping your chin by your chest, tuck your pelvis to roll along your back one vertebra at a time, stopping when you reach the bottoms of your shoulders. Then roll back up, stopping when your legs are extended into the "V."

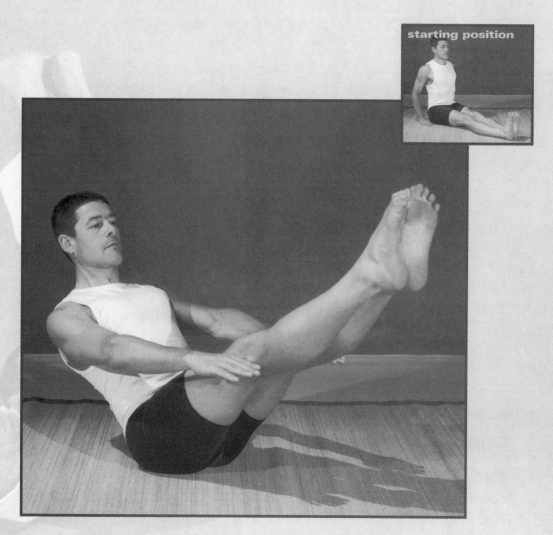
starting position

GETTING INTO POSE: Begin in Staff Pose (page 31). Inhale and place your hands lightly behind your head. Exhale and lean back to find your balance point (about 45 degrees) while lifting your legs toward the ceiling 45 degrees. Keep your legs straight and lengthen your lower back to prevent your back from sagging. Inhale and reach your hands forward, thumbside up, so that your wrists are next to your knees.

Hold for 5 breaths.

Bharadvaja's Pose I
(Bharadvajasana I)

■ Bharadvaja = one of seven seers ■ (bah-ROD-va-JAHS-anna) ■

GENERAL BENEFITS: Stretches the neck, shoulders, arms, chest, hips, and spine; releases the arches of the feet

VARIATION: Reach the back of your right hand toward the left side of your back as you turn your head to gaze over your left shoulder.

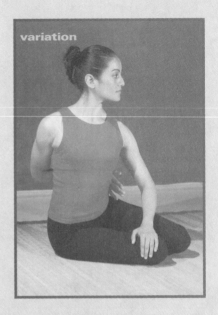
variation

Martial arts application

BENEFITS: Releases shoulder, back, and hip tension from rolls and falls

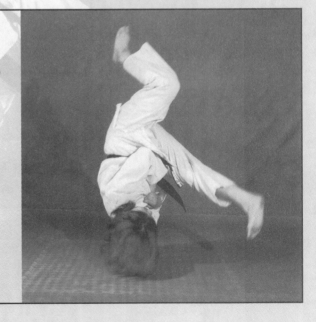

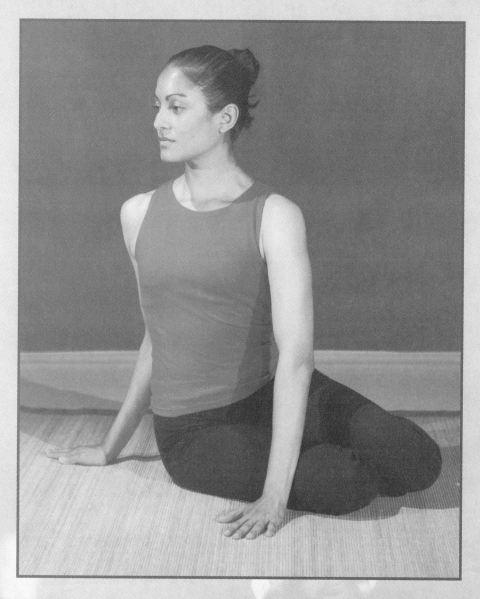

GETTING INTO POSE: Sit with your knees bent in front of you and your feet flat on the floor. Drop your knees to your right, letting your feet slide toward your left hip so your left ankle rests in your right arch. Keeping your torso vertical, lift out of your waist and twist your torso and head to your right. Place your left hand on or next to your right knee and your right hand on the floor behind your right hip, toward your spine. Gaze over your right shoulder.

Hold for 5 breaths, then gaze over your left shoulder and hold for 5 more breaths. Repeat on the other side.

Locust (Salabhasana)

■ *salabha* = locust ■ (sha-la-BAHS-anna) ■

GENERAL BENEFITS: Strengthens the back, butt, hamstrings, and arms; stretches the shoulders, chest, stomach, and thighs

Martial arts application

BENEFITS: Releases shoulder, abdominal, and back tension from rolls and some falls; strengthens the arms for slapping and/or supporting weight

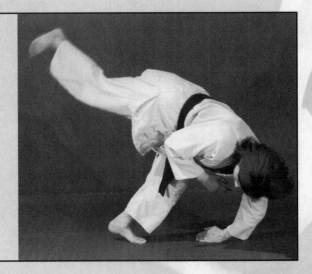

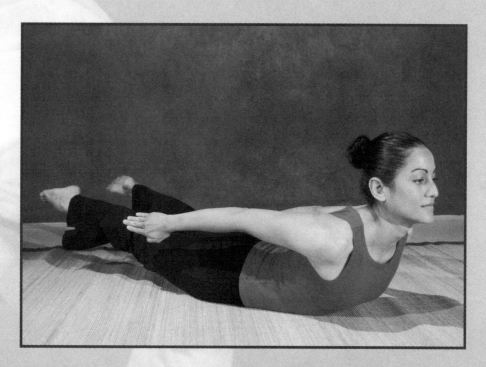

GETTING INTO POSE: Lie face down, chin on the floor, with your arms alongside your body, palms up, and your legs extended. Inhale then exhale to simultaneously raise your head, chest, arms, and legs off the floor. Keep your arms parallel to the floor and your neck long. Reach your fingertips and toes behind you.

Hold for 5 breaths.

Camel (Ustrasana)

■ *ustra* = camel ■ (oosh-TRAHS-anna) ■

GENERAL BENEFITS: Strengthens the back; stretches the shoulders, chest, stomach, quads, hip flexors, and ankles

VARIATION: Press your insteps into the floor.

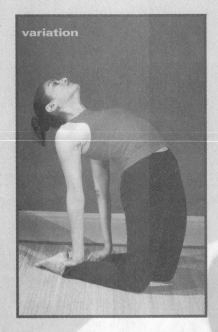

variation

Martial arts application

BENEFITS: Releases shoulder, abdominal, arm, and back tension from rolls and some falls

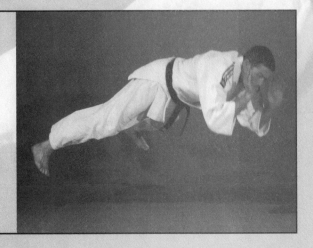

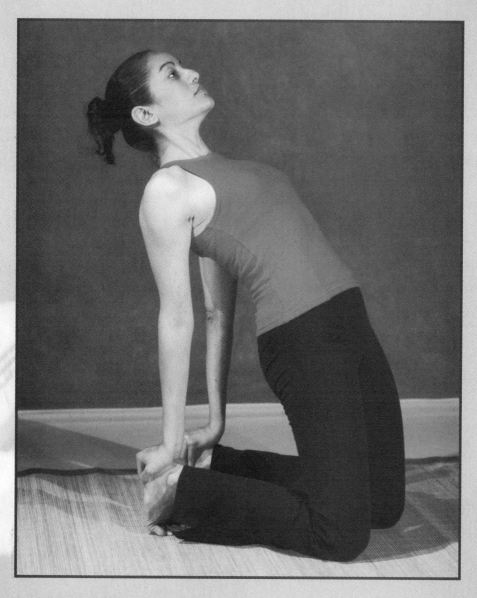

GETTING INTO POSE: Kneel with your knees directly under your hips and your toes tucked under. Place your palms on your lower back. Inhale and lift your chest by extending out from your waist. Exhale and slowly arch back, releasing one hand at a time to your heels. Keep your head in line with your spine, drawing your shoulders away from your ears. Lift your hips forward, lengthening your abs.

Hold for 5 breaths.

Plow (Halasana)

■ *hala* = plow ■ (hah-LAHS-anna) ■

GENERAL BENEFITS: Stretches the shoulders and spine

MODIFICATION: For additional support, with your elbows firmly on the floor, place your hands on your lower back.

Martial arts application

BENEFITS: Relieves the impact to the spine, shoulders, and neck from rolling/falling; stretches the muscles used in back rolls

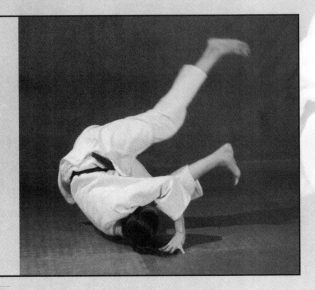

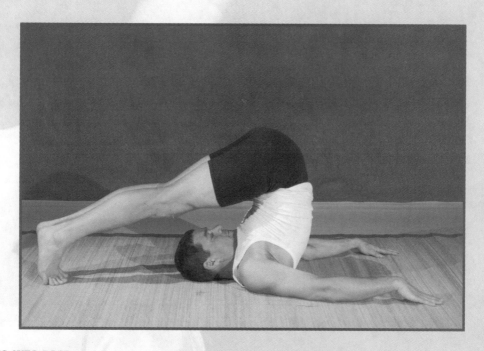

GETTING INTO POSE: Lie on your back with your arms along your sides, knees bent and feet on the floor. Exhale and bring your knees to your chest, extending your legs back and over your head to lift your hips up. Place your arms along the floor. Continue extending your legs until your toes reach the floor, using your upper back as the base so as not to flatten your neck.

Hold for 10 breaths.

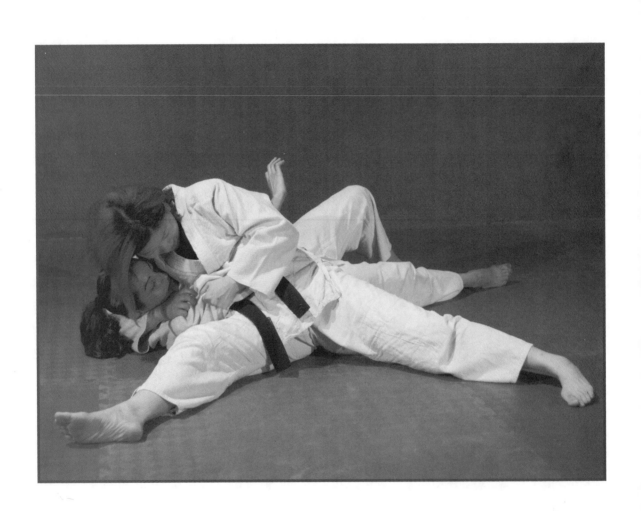

Grappling

Grappling is far more than simply rolling around on the ground, trying to crush your partner using brute force and sheer weight. It involves complex mind and body coordination to maneuver around a partner who's also moving—you're vying for the ideal position to execute a pin, lock, choke, or other submission technique before your partner does the same. The dynamic nature of grappling requires body and spatial awareness and enough flexibility to evade holds and avoid injury.

KEY ANATOMY

There is no part of your body that isn't used—whether deliberately or accidentally—to apply or evade a technique. Grappling is truly a full-body workout.

Essential Elements

BODY AWARENESS/CONTROL One of the main goals in grappling is to manipulate your partner into a position that lets you apply a submission technique (such as a hold, choke, or joint lock) that will either elicit a tap-out (submission) or control your opponent for a prescribed length of time. Knowing where your body is at all times is crucial on several levels. Once you have your partner in an auspicious position, you have milliseconds to assess where your hand or hip needs to go in order to effectively apply a technique. Body placement is important when executing techniques: if his shoulder is too low, you won't get an arm bar; if you turn

his hand over too far, you've lost your wrist lock; or if your butt is too high when you're trying to pin him, you may suddenly find yourself being rolled onto your back.

From a defense standpoint, body awareness helps you evade submission techniques attempted by your partner: knowing where your body is at all times prevents you from (among other things) exposing an arm or leg to attack, and prevents you from being involuntarily flipped over or thrown when your weight is distributed poorly.

Manipulating your partner's body and applying submission techniques is not

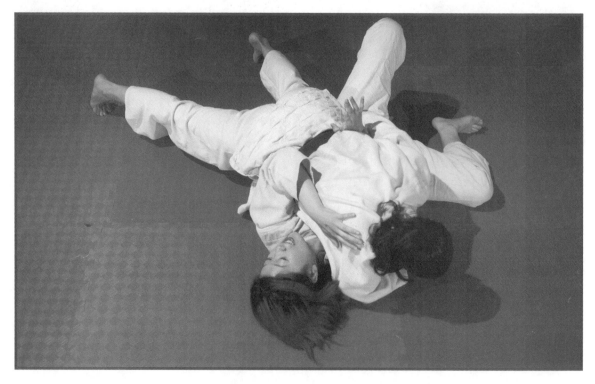

The Martial Artist's Book of Yoga

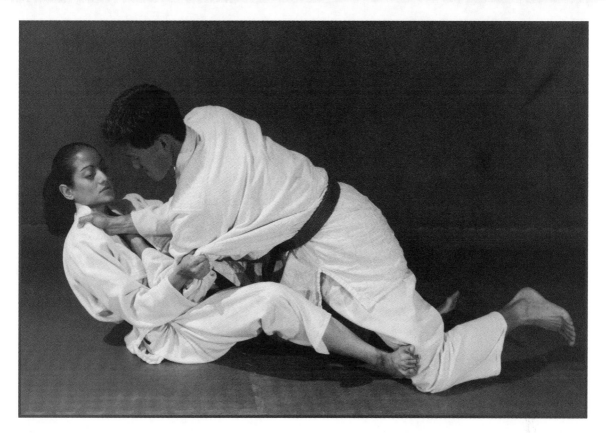

simply a function of your arms—your legs and hips play key roles. Being aware and in control of your body lets you move all parts as a coherent unit, and lets you apply exactly the amount of force you need to get the desired response. Awareness also helps you determine when yielding to a technique rather than resisting can actually improve your position.

FLEXIBILITY Doing the splits is not essential to being a good grappler. However, flexibility is what lets you squirm out of pins and joint locks and escape pretzel-like situations. Flexible legs and hips are useful in hooking around your partner's head/neck to keep her in check. Most importantly, flexibility is the key to preventing and reducing strain and/or injury from inadvertent exertion, such as when you find yourself suddenly rolling over your neck or your legs being pried wide apart.

Benefits of Yoga

The Fundamental poses improve grappling skills by strengthening your legs and improving range of motion in your hips and spine—all important for maneuvering on the ground and controlling your partner. Since grappling uses your entire body, the poses in this section address all your many body parts and functions. They encourage flexibility in your joints—particularly in your neck and back—so they are more resistant to injuries. The poses promote ease of movement, restoring muscular balance by stretching and releasing muscles tight from overuse, strain, or natural inflexibility. Many of these poses involve twisting and turning both your upper and lower body, increasing your awareness of your body positioning while improving body control. In addition, this twisting enhances spine mobility, important for wriggling around on the ground.

Poses for Grappling

Bound Angle (*Baddha Konasana*)

Cowface (*Gomukhasana*)

Half Lord of the Fishes (*Ardha Matsyendrasana*)

Hero (*Virasana*)

Bow (*Dhanurasana*)

Bridge (*Setu Bandha Sarvangasana*)

All-Limb (*Sarvangasana*)

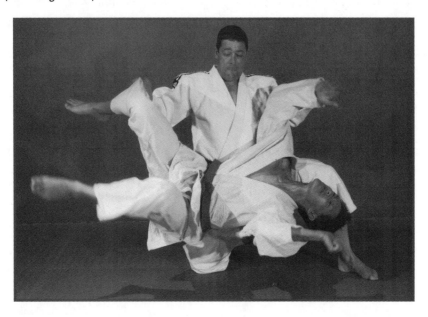

Other Poses

These poses that appear elsewhere in the book also benefit grappling moves:

Bharadvaja's Pose I *(page 44)*: warms up and releases the spine and major joints used in grappling

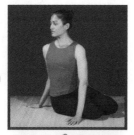

Plow *(page 50)*: improves spine and shoulder flexibility; teaches control from an inverted position

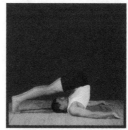

Gate *(page 40)*: reverses the compressing effects of grappling

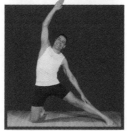

Front Extension *(page 82)*: reverses the compressing effects of grappling; strengthens the arms for maneuvering

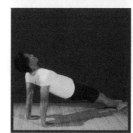

Happy Mountain *(page 84)*: conditions the upper body for grappling

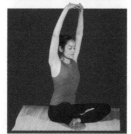

Seated Angle *(page 106):* stretches the lower body; strengthens the back

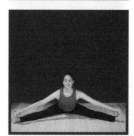

Lotus *(page 86)*: conditions the lower body for grappling

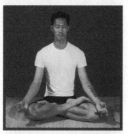

Locust *(page 46)*: strengthens the arms for maneuvering; reverses the compressing effects of grappling

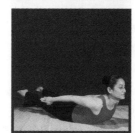

One-Legged King Pigeon *(page 104):* stretches the lower body

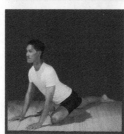

Crane *(page 120):* strengthens the arms for maneuvering; teaches balance and even weight distribution

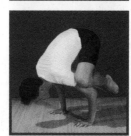

Bound Angle (Baddha Konasana)

■ *baddha* = bound; *kona* = angle ■ (BAH-dah cone-AHS-anna) ■

GENERAL BENEFITS: Stretches the inner thighs, groin muscles, knees, back, and hips; strengthens the back; opens the hips

VARIATION: From sitting upright, fold at your hips and reach your arms forward on the floor, bringing your chest to your hands and your forehead to the floor.

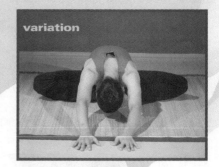
variation

Martial arts application

BENEFITS: Prepares the hips for control and transitional movements that use the legs

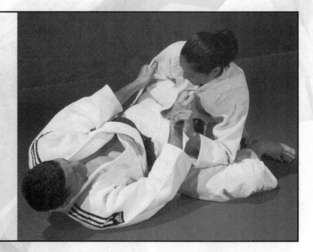

The Martial Artist's Book of Yoga

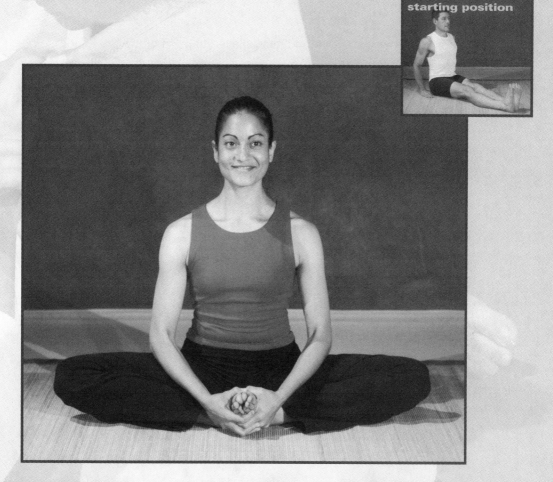

starting position

GETTING INTO POSE: Begin in Staff Pose (page 31). Bend your knees to press the soles of your feet together. Wrap your hands around your feet and draw your heels in toward your pubis. Lift your chest, rolling your shoulders back and down to straighten your spine. Let your knees release to the floor.

Hold for 10 breaths.

Cowface (Gomukhasana)

■ *go* = cow; *mukha* = face ■ (go-moo-KAHS-anna) ■

GENERAL BENEFITS: Stretches the shoulders, arms, wrists, ankles, hips, and quads; opens the shoulders

MODIFICATION: If you cannot hook your fingers, place the palm of the top hand on your upper back and reach for your lower hand.

Martial arts application

BENEFITS: Warms up and releases the major joints used in grappling

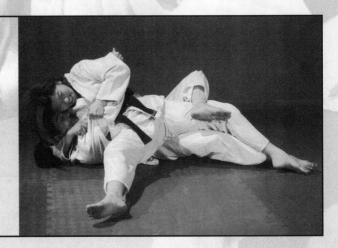

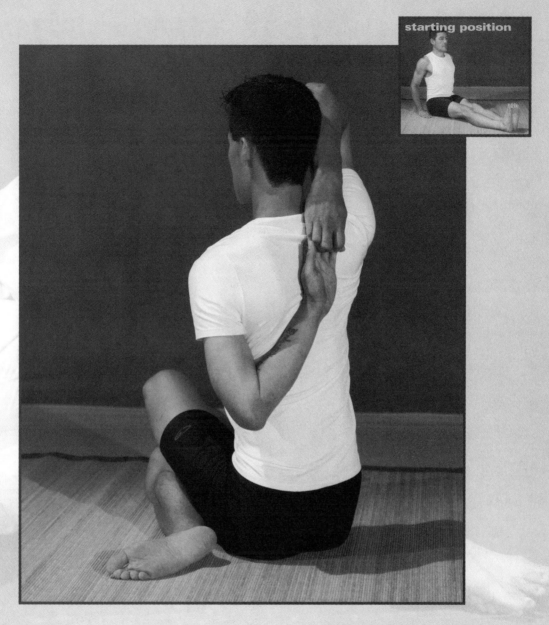

starting position

GETTING INTO POSE: Begin in Staff Pose (page 31). Bend your knees to place your feet on the floor. Slide your right foot under the left knee to the outside of your left hip. Cross your left knee over the right to bring your left foot to the outside of your right hip. Keeping the top of your head lifting toward the ceiling, place the back of your left hand on your back, fingers pointing to the ceiling. Raise your right arm to the ceiling, then slide your hand down your back to hook the fingers of your left hand.

Hold for 10 breaths. Repeat on the other side.

Half Lord of the Fishes
(Ardha Matsyendrasana)

■ *ardha* = half; *matsya* = fish; *indra* = ruler ■ (AR-dah MOT-see-en-DRAHS-anna) ■

GENERAL BENEFITS: Stretches the neck, shoulders, spine, and hips

Martial arts application

BENEFITS: Prepares the spine and hips for twisting movements

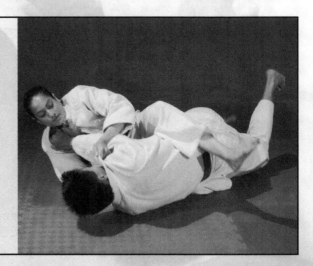

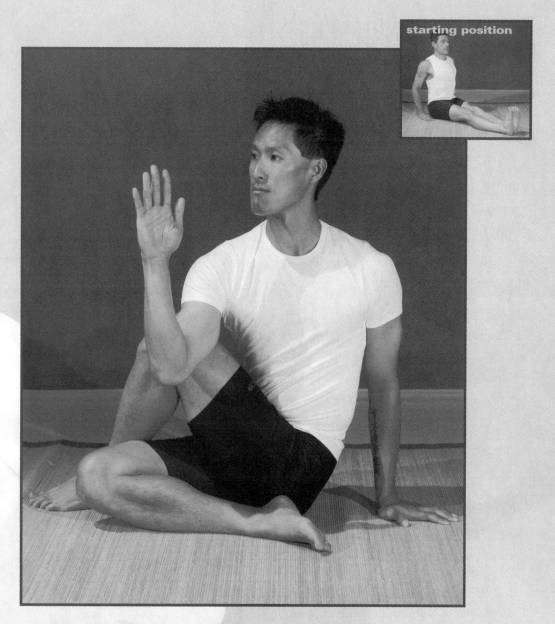

GETTING INTO POSE: Begin in Staff Pose (page 31). Bend your left knee toward your chest and place your left foot on the outside of your right thigh. Slide your right foot under your left buttock. Place the back of your right arm against the outside of your left knee; bend your left elbow so that your fingers point up and your forearm is perpendicular to the floor. Press your left hand into the floor behind your spine and twist from your tailbone to press your right triceps against the outside of your left knee. Gaze over your right shoulder.

Hold for 5 breaths, then gaze over your left shoulder and hold for 5 more breaths. Repeat on the other side.

Hero (Virasana)

■ *vira* = man, hero ■ (veer-AHS-anna) ■

GENERAL BENEFITS: Stretches the quads, knees, ankles, and insteps; strengthens the arches

MODIFICATION: If your butt does not reach the floor, sit on a blanket or book placed between your feet for elevation and support.

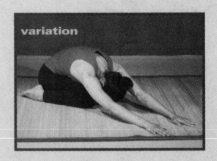
variation

VARIATION: Fold forward from your hips, bringing your belly then chest to your thighs.

ADVANCED VARIATION (RECLINING HERO): From sitting upright, exhale and lower your back toward the floor, placing your hands, then forearms, then elbows down behind you. Finally, rest your back on the floor, arms out to the sides with your palms up. Push into your forearms to get up. *CAUTION: Do not do this variation if your butt does not rest easily on the floor.*

Martial arts application

BENEFITS: If you draw your heels together, raise your butt, and rise onto the balls of your feet, you'll find yourself in a common grappling position. This pose trains even weight distribution when in a mount position.

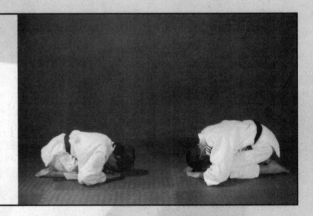

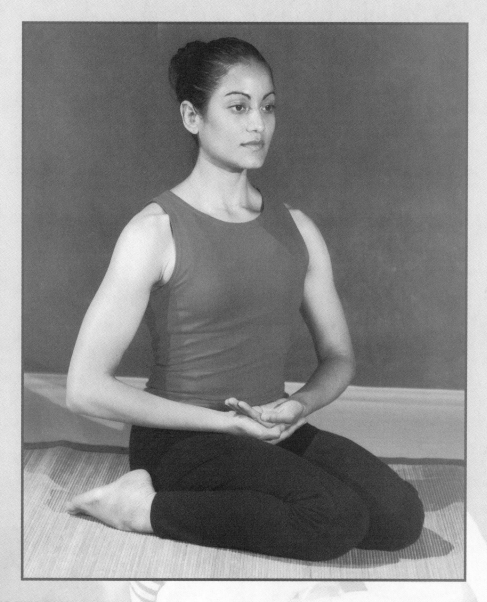

GETTING INTO POSE: Start by sitting on your heels, with the tops of your feet on the floor and your torso upright. Keeping your knees together, slowly slide your feet apart until they're just wider than your hips. Lower your butt to the floor. Roll your shoulders back and down and rest your hands in your lap or on your thighs.

Hold for 10 breaths.

Bow (Dhanurasana)

■ *dhanu* = bow ■ (don-your-AHS-anna) ■

GENERAL BENEFITS: Stretches the stomach, chest, throat, quads, hip flexors, groin muscles, and ankles; strengthens the back

Martial arts application

BENEFITS: Reverses the compressing effect of the defensive fetal or turtle position

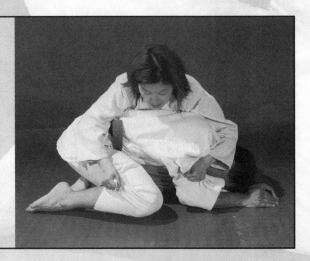

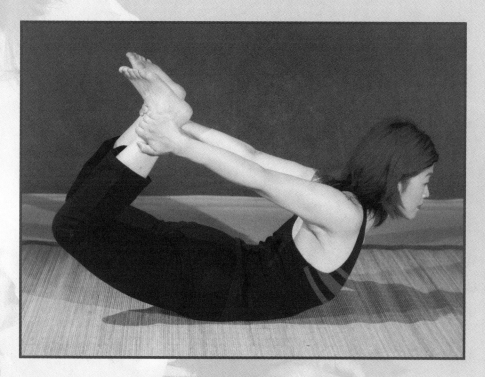

GETTING INTO POSE: Start by lying on your stomach with your belly in and firm; rest your arms along your sides, palms up. Exhale and bend you knees to bring your heels to your butt. Grasp your ankles and reach your legs away from your butt, letting your thighs, chest, and head lift off the floor.

Hold for 10 breaths.

Bridge (Setu Bandha Sarvangasana)

■ *setu* = bridge; *bandha* = lock; *sarva* = all; *anga* = limb ■
(SET-too BAHN-dah sar-van-GAHS-anna) ■

GENERAL BENEFITS: Stretches the chest, neck, shoulders, and spine; strengthens the quads and knees

Martial arts application

BENEFITS: Strengthens the movement used to dismount a partner who's straddling you when you're on your back

CHALLENGE: Move your arms to the sides and, keeping your knees and feet in place, lower and lift your hips 10 times.

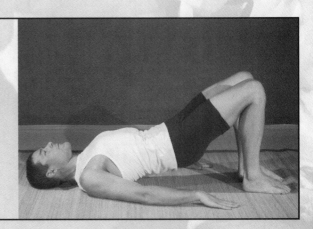

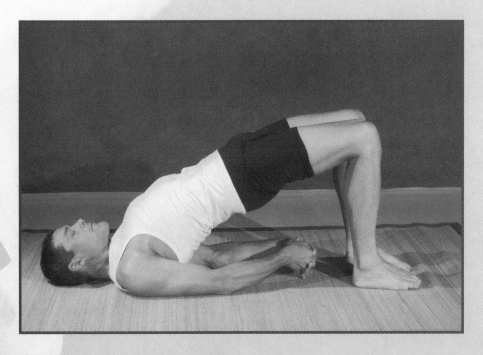

GETTING INTO POSE: Begin by lying on your back with your arms along your sides. Bend your knees and bring your heels close to your butt. Pressing into your arms and feet, roll from your tailbone and up along your spine to raise your hips to knee height. Pull your shoulder blades toward each other and reach your hands, which are clasped together on the floor beneath your pelvis, toward your feet.

Hold for 10 breaths.

All-Limb (Sarvangasana)

■ *sarva* = all; *anga* = limb ■ (sar-van-GAHS-anna) ■

Also known as **Shoulder Stand**

GENERAL BENEFITS: Stretches the shoulders and spine; teaches balance

Martial arts application

BENEFITS: Improves control from an inverted position

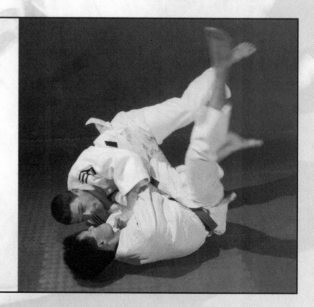

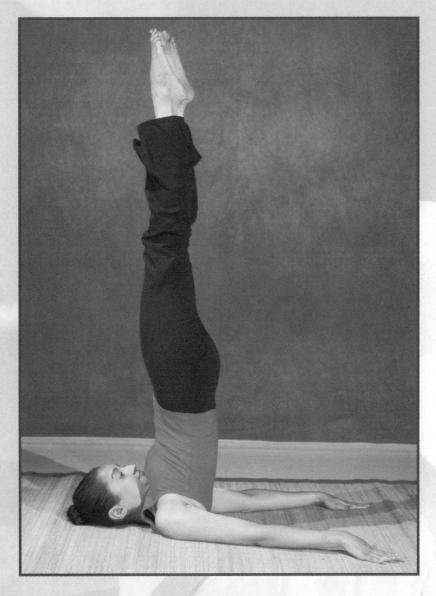

GETTING INTO POSE: Lie on your back with your arms along your sides. Bend your knees and bring your heels close to your butt. Exhale and round your back to bring your knees to your chest. Continue bringing your knees toward your ears and shoulders until you can place your hands on your lower back for support, keeping your elbows in and your upper arms pressed into the floor. Inhale then exhale, unfolding your legs toward the ceiling so that they are perpendicular to the floor. If you feel balanced, release your arms to the floor.

Hold for 5 breaths.

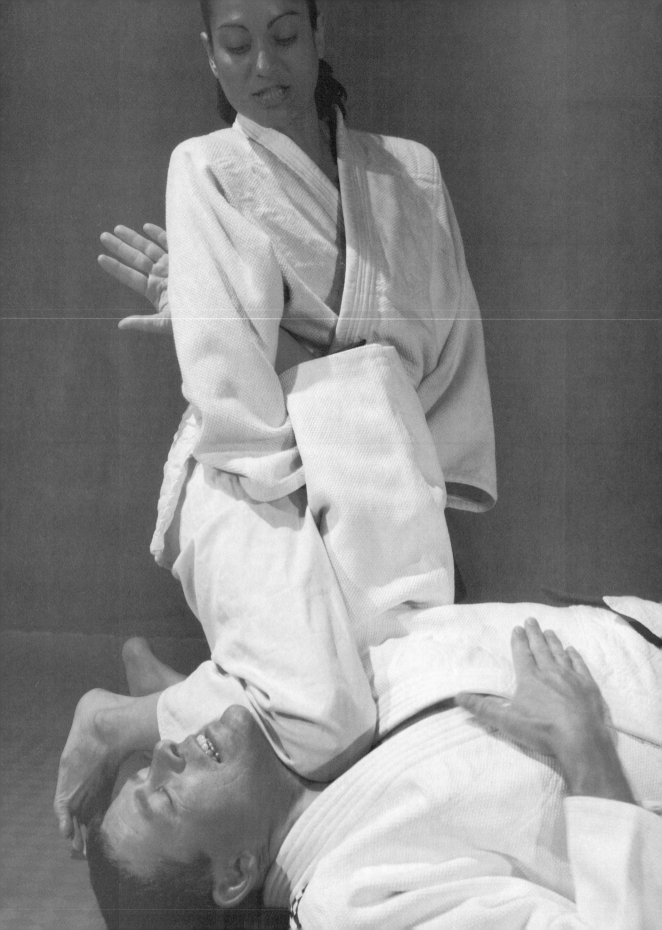

Joint Locks

Martial arts styles such as jujitsu, hapkido, and aikido implement these often-subtle but powerful techniques as forms of self-defense and/or control of an opponent. Locks involve isolating a joint and forcing it to move in an unnatural direction. Elbows, fingers, and knees can be hyperextended until they're on the verge of breaking, and ankles, toes, shoulders, fingers, and wrists can be bent or twisted to elicit debilitating pain or immobilize an opponent.

KEY ANATOMY

No joints are immune from being locked: fingers, toes, ankles, wrists, knees, shoulders, elbows. From standing, locks can be applied by a combination of fingers, hands, and forearms, with the torso providing the bulk of the power. In other situations, such as grappling, legs and elbows can also be utilized as fulcrums or levers.

BODY AWARENESS/CONTROL Since applying effective joint locks requires the precise placement of fulcrums and levers and an exact amount of pressure, every movement leading up to the actual technique counts. When you're performing a joint lock, body awareness is critical in helping you determine when your body is just the right distance from your partner, with your feet placed just so (if you're standing); that your elbows are close to your hips so your technique derives power from the movement of your entire body, not just your arms and hands; that you don't over- or underrotate the selected joint and/or apply pressure to the wrong point. With awareness comes the ability to control (or begin to control) all these many movements so the end result is a well-executed technique resulting in a lock or hold of your opponent. When you have true control, you can also accurately gauge exactly the amount of force you need.

BALANCE Footwork is integral to performing an effective joint lock, whether you intend to control the fingers/wrists/etc. or shuttle a resisting person from point A to point B once you've applied the lock. Good balance lets you step or duck into position smoothly and quickly

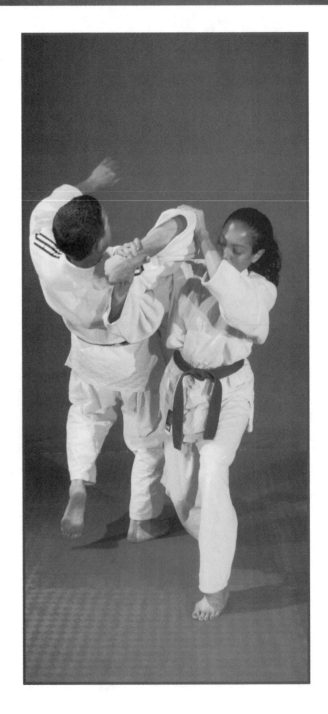

so you don't lose the ligament tightness you've secured, and it lets you effectively transfer the power from your body's movement to your opponent's joints.

FLEXIBILITY It seems logical that receivers of joint locks should be more concerned about flexibility than those who apply the locks. Repeated trauma to joints often results in soreness and tight- ness in connecting tissue, sometimes in strains or sprains. Flexibility is the key to keeping these tissues healthy and resilient. At the same time, joint flexibility is beneficial for applying joint locks as well: relaxed shoulders and hands enjoy increased range of motion, while a loose back and hips generate more speed and power than their stiffer counterparts.

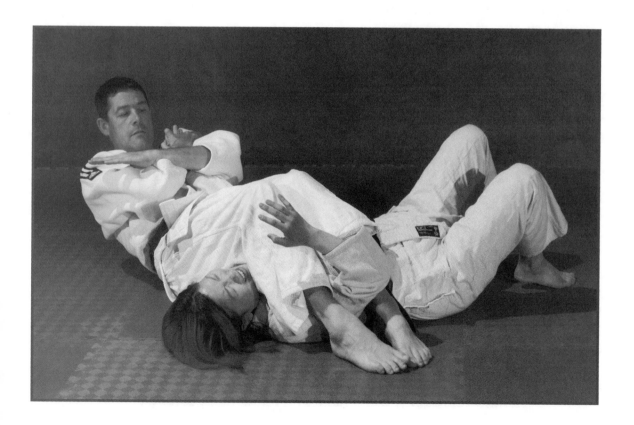

Benefits of Yoga

The poses in the Fundamentals section all help improve the execution of joint locks by strengthening proper stances and improving balance and the body's ability to work as one unit. When you practice an art that includes joint locks in its repertoire, you tend to receive your share of pain. The poses in this section address the physical wear and tear receivers of joint locks endure, by stretching, releasing, and aligning the muscles/tendons/ligaments around the joints and increasing/restoring flexibility to tight muscles, including the back. This increased range of motion helps you apply the techniques more fluidly and effectively as well—but these yoga poses particularly help improve resistance to injury and pain.

Poses for Joint Locks

Prayer (*Namaste*)

Intense Leg Extension III (*Padottanasana III*)

Front Extension (*Purvottanasana*)

Happy Mountain (*Sukha Parvatasana*)

Lotus (*Padmasana*)

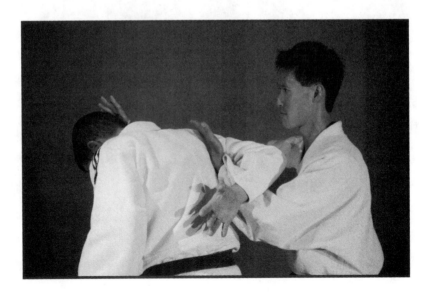

The Martial Artist's Book of Yoga

Other Poses

These poses that appear elsewhere in the book also benefit joint locks:

Bharadvaja's Pose I *(page 44)*: improves hip and spine mobility

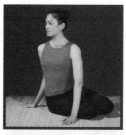

Gate *(page 40)*: stretches the hips and the sides of the body

Camel *(page 48)*: promotes spine flexibility; stretches the arms, shoulders, and chest

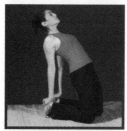

Locust *(page 46)*: stretches the shoulders; strengthens the spine, legs, and arms

Cowface *(page 60)*: stretches the major joints; prepares the shoulders for locks

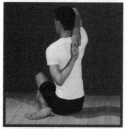

Sideways Extension *(page 96)*: prepares the wrists and shoulders for locks

Eagle *(page 132)*: stretches the hips, arms, and shoulders; teaches balance

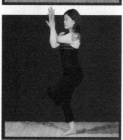

One-Legged Downward-Facing Dog *(page 122)*: strengthens the arms, wrists, shoulders, and back

Four-Limbed Staff *(page 114)*: strengthens the arms, wrists, and shoulders

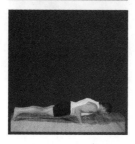

Vasishta's Pose *(page 116)*: strengthens the arms and wrists; improves wrist flexibility

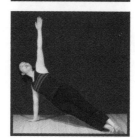

Prayer (Namaste)

■ *namaste* = "I bow to you" ■ (NAH-muh-stay) ■

GENERAL BENEFITS: Stretches the shoulders, chest, forearms, wrists, and hands

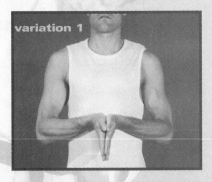

VARIATION 1: Keeping your forearms in place, turn your hands down to touch your pinkies to your belly.

VARIATION 2: Bring both hands, fingers up, behind your back and press your palms together.

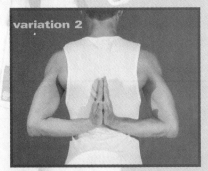

Martial arts application

BENEFITS: Reverses the effects of wrist locks

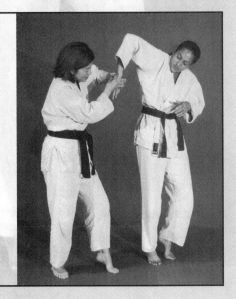

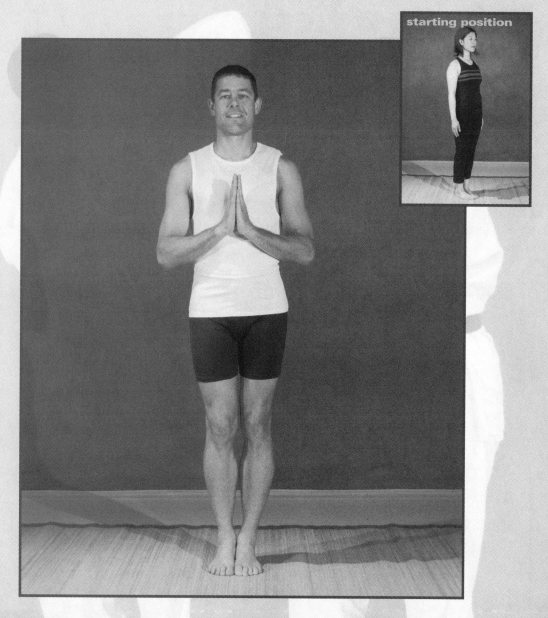

GETTING INTO POSE: Begin in Mountain Pose (page 27). Bring both thumbs to your sternum and press your palms together. Keeping your shoulders back, your fingers pointing up, and the heels of your palms together, lift your ribs and chest and draw your forearms parallel to the floor.

Hold for 10 breaths.

Intense Leg Extension III (Padottanasana III)

■ *pada* = leg; *ut* = intense; *tan* = to stretch or extend ■
(pah-doh-tahn-AHS-anna) ■

GENERAL BENEFITS: Stretches the hamstrings, spine, hips, and shoulders; releases the neck

Martial arts application

BENEFITS: Improves shoulders' ability to endure locks

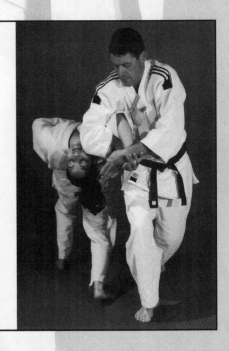

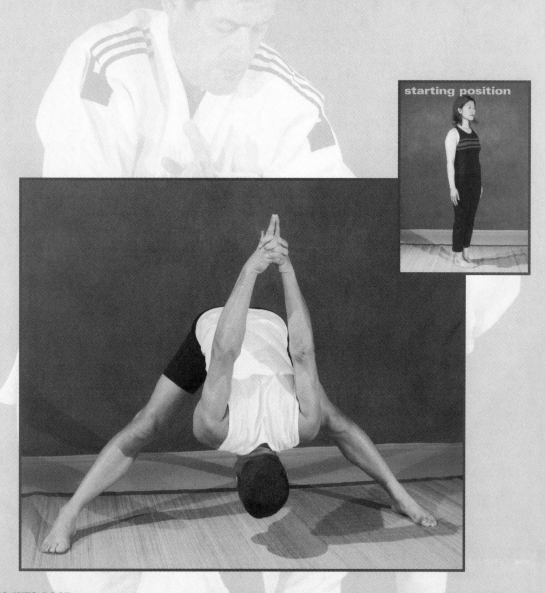

starting position

GETTING INTO POSE: Begin in Mountain Pose (page 27). Step your feet wide apart and place your hands on your hips. Inhale and, extending from your waist, reach your chest forward. Exhale and, hinging from your hips, reach your torso toward your legs. Press your palms together behind you and interlock your fingers, then press your hands toward the ceiling.

Hold for 5 breaths. Switch the clasp of your hands and hold for 5 more breaths.

Front Extension (Purvottanasana)

■ *purvo* = front of the body; *tan* = to stretch or extend ■ (pur-voh-tahn-AHS-anna) ■

Also known as **Inclined Plane** *or* **Reverse Plank**

GENERAL BENEFITS: Strengthens the arms, shoulders, wrists, and legs; stretches the hands, wrists, arms, shoulders, chest, ankles, and feet

Martial arts application

BENEFITS: Improves shoulders', wrists', and ankles' ability to endure locks

CHALLENGE: Lower the hips to the floor, then raise them back up. Repeat this lower and lift 4 more times.

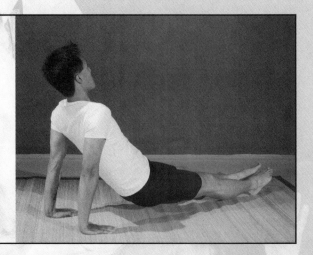

The Martial Artist's Book of Yoga

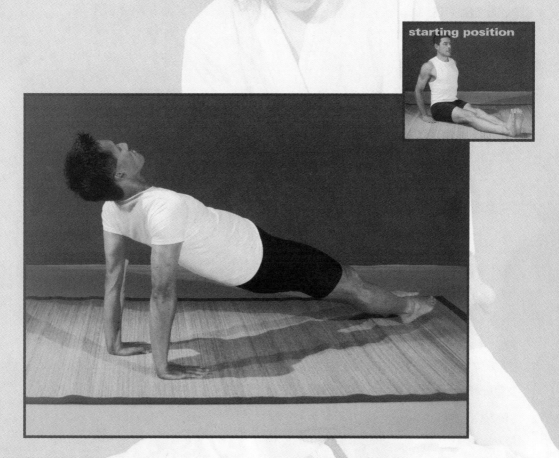

starting position

GETTING INTO POSE: Begin in Staff Pose (page 31). Move your hands about six inches back from your hips, keeping your forearms perpendicular to the floor. Pressing your hands firmly into the floor, lengthen your arms and lift your hips toward the ceiling. Draw your kneecaps toward your hips, press into the heels of your feet, and reach your toes to the floor. Your body should form one straight line from toes to ears.

Hold for 5 breaths.

Happy Mountain
(Sukha Parvatasana)

■ *sukha* = joy; *parvata* = mountain ■ (soo-KAH par-vah-TAHS-anna) ■

GENERAL BENEFITS: Stretches the fingers, hands, wrists, arms, shoulders, and spine

VARIATIONS: This can also be done in Half Lotus (page 86), Lotus (page 86), and Hero (page 64).

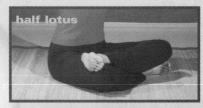

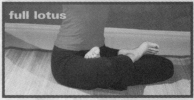

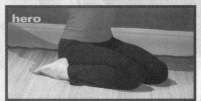

Martial arts application

BENEFITS: Reverses the effects of wrist and finger locks; improves shoulders' ability to endure locks

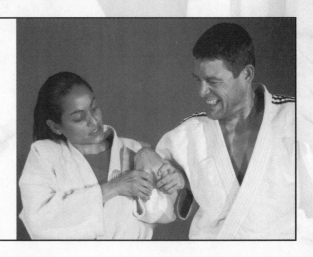

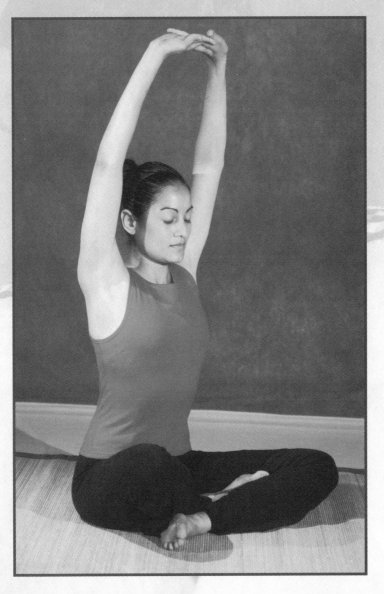

GETTING INTO POSE: Sit in a comfortable cross-legged position. Imagine that a string is pulling the top of your head to the ceiling. Place your hands in your lap, palms up, and interlace your fingers. Inhale, then exhale as you extend your arms above your head with your biceps by your ears, turning your palms to face the ceiling. Keep your shoulders down.

Hold for 5 breaths. Switch the clasp of your hands and repeat for 5 more breaths.

Lotus (Padmasana)

■ *padma* = lotus ■ (pod-MAHS-anna) ■

GENERAL BENEFITS: Stretches the quads, knees, ankles, and insteps

MODIFICATION (HALF LOTUS): Place only one foot on the thigh at a time.

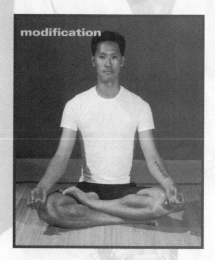

modification

Martial arts application

BENEFITS: Improves resistance to ankle locks

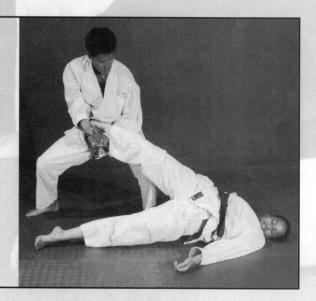

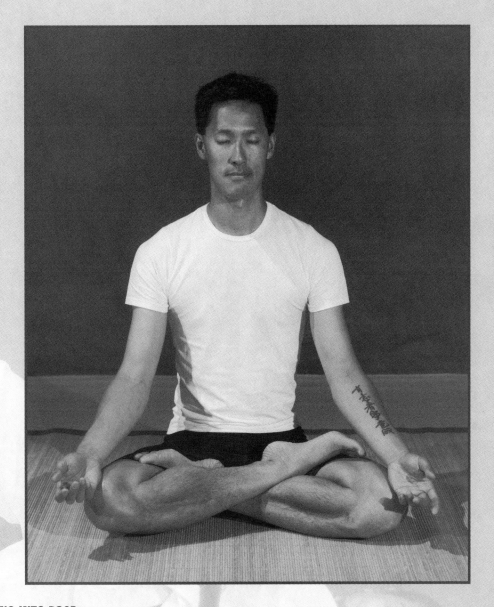

GETTING INTO POSE: Sit in a comfortable cross-legged position. Take your left foot and place it on top of your right thigh, then take your right foot and place it on top of your left thigh. Rest the backs of your hands on your knees.

Hold for 5 breaths. Repeat the process by starting with your right foot first.

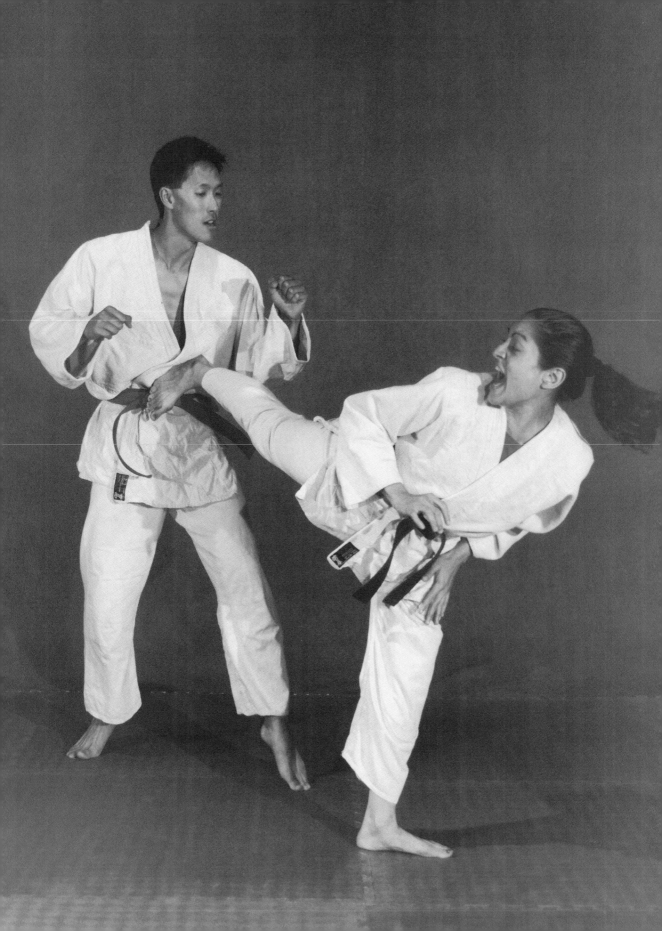

Anyone can bend their knee and extend their leg to punt a ball or dance like a Rockette. But the versatile offensive techniques executed in martial arts like karate, taekwondo, and kung fu require instruction and practice before they can be delivered safely, powerfully, efficiently, and accurately. Whether you do butterfly kicks, shin stomps, axe kicks to the head, or spinning hook kicks, you must have a healthy combination of flexibility, balance, and body control/alignment. Even "simple" stretch kicks, performed to warm up the legs and back before executing formal kicks, can be challenging if you're not properly prepared.

KEY ANATOMY

The hips, legs, and feet are the major components of a kick. The abdominals and lower back also play significant roles.

Essential Elements

BODY AWARENESS/CONTROL/ALIGNMENT

Kicks require you to pick up your knee, turn over your hip, and extend your leg. These gross motor movements are achieved fairly easily, but the finer details essential for good form and function (angling your foot and toes properly, not hunching over in an attempt to kick higher than you're able to) come with the awareness and control that eventually result from practice. Awareness also helps you control extraneous and often inhibiting movements that waste energy and/or slow down or reduce power in kicks: tensing your shoulders, flailing or counter-torquing your arms as you twist into a kick. Extra control is needed for turning or spinning kicks, since overrotation throws you off balance and underrotation stops the kick short of its intended target. As you gain control of your body's movements, you can better align your toes, feet, hips, and legs for optimal performance. Together, good body control and alignment help you kick with power, accurately strike your targets, and avoid injuries that misuse of muscles, tendons, and ligaments might cause.

BALANCE

Since all kicks require picking up at least one leg off the floor, balance is critical in keeping you from toppling over. It also prevents you from twisting your ankle or torquing your knee as you

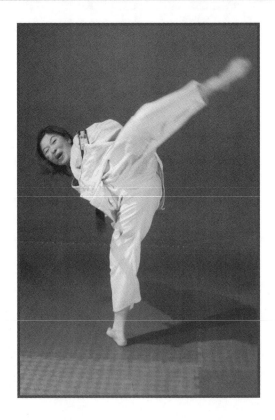

set your foot/feet down afterward. The issue of balance becomes even more crucial if you practice turning or spinning kicks—movements that involve rotating on the ball of the foot, twisting the torso, and extending the leg. Coupled with body control and alignment, good balance quickens and smooths out your footwork for faster kicks and quicker recovery.

FLEXIBILITY

The flexibility of your legs, hips, and spine determines how high and fast you can kick. The more flexible you are, the greater range of motion you have: your axe kick strikes higher targets, your front kick covers more distance. Flexible muscles and joints also let you chamber, extend, and retract your kicks much more quickly—you deliver them more explosively and recover with greater agility, so you can execute your next kick faster.

BREATH CONTROL You've likely been taught to *kihap/kiai* ("spirit yell") as you land a kick. This is not simply to call attention to your technique. The action of exhaling explosively, regardless of volume, serves to focus all your internal energy (*chi* or *ki*) into the kick. The synchronization of kick and *kihap* results in more powerful techniques. Learning to control your breath has other advantages as well, such as better aerobic capacity and delivery of oxygen to muscles.

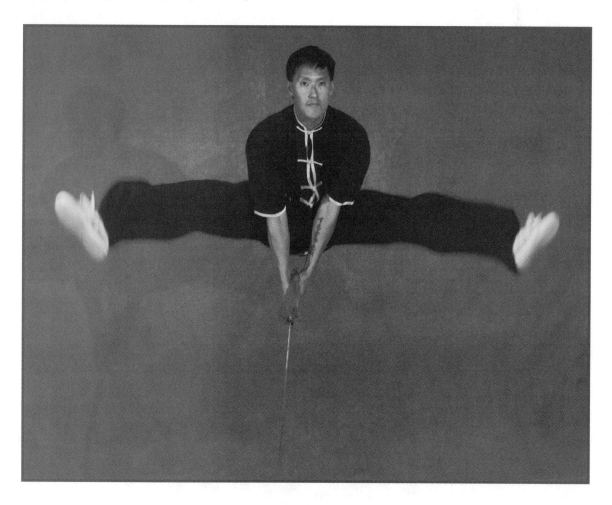

Benefits of Yoga

The Fundamental poses benefit your kicks by promoting proper alignment and strengthening and stretching your hips and spine. The poses in this section all encourage flexibility by taking your joints (namely your hips, knees, and ankles) through their full range of motion and by stretching tight muscles and releasing those that have been overused (such as the quadriceps and hip flexors). They also promote proper anatomical alignment, which further improves joint and muscle function. The one-legged and revolved poses challenge your balance and body control as they simultaneously strengthen your legs and core muscles.

Poses for Kicks

Tree (*Vrksasana*)

Sideways Extension (*Parsvottanasana*)

Half Moon (*Ardha Chandrasana*)

Warrior III (*Virabhadrasana III*)

Reverse Triangle (*Parivrtta Trikonasana*)

One-Legged King Pigeon (*Eka Pada Rajakapotasana*)

Seated Angle (*Upavishta Konasana*)

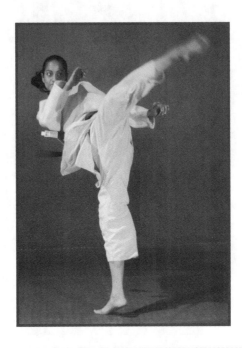

The Martial Artist's Book of Yoga

Other Poses

These poses that appear elsewhere in the book are also beneficial for kicks:

Bound Angle *(page 58)*: stretches the groin muscles

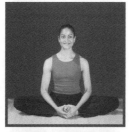

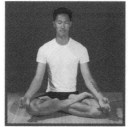

Lotus *(page 86)*: stretches the lower body

Camel *(page 48)*: stretches the quads; releases the hip flexors

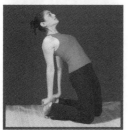

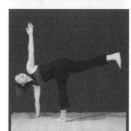

Reverse Half Moon *(page 134)*: strengthens the legs and ankles; teaches balance; promotes spine and hip flexibility

Half Lord of the Fishes *(page 62):* promotes hip and spine flexibility

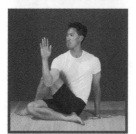

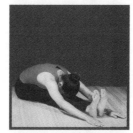

Intense Stretch of the West *(page 138)*: stretches the hamstrings for improved range of motion in linear kicks

Hero *(page 64)*: stretches the lower body

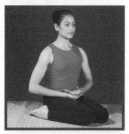

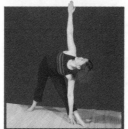

Triangle *(page 118)*: reverses the compressing effect of side and roundhouse kicks

Locust *(page 46)*: strengthens the quads, hamstrings, and butt; reverses hunched-over posture

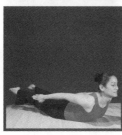

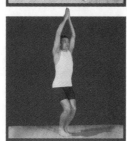

Powerful *(page 130)*: strengthens the knees, quads, and ankles

Tree (Vrksasana)

■ *vrksa* = tree ■ (vrik-SHAHS-anna) ■

GENERAL BENEFITS: Improves balance; stretches and strengthens the legs, groin muscles, and feet; opens the hips; strengthens the ankles; lengthens the spine

MODIFICATION: If balance is difficult, try this standing next to a wall or chair.

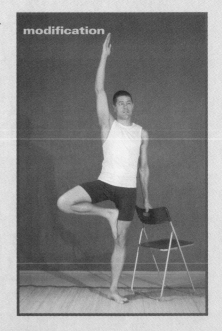

modification

Martial arts application

BENEFITS: Improves balance for all kicks, including turning/spinning versions; improves range of motion for roundhouse, split, and butterfly kicks

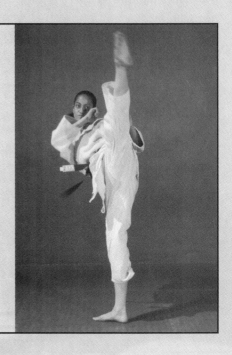

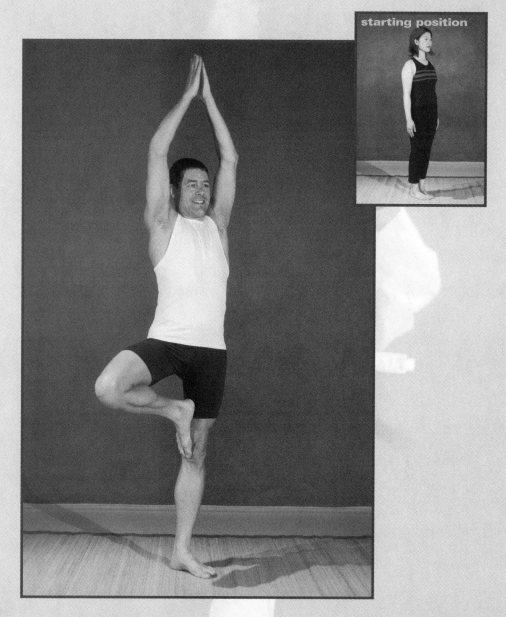

starting position

GETTING INTO POSE: Begin in Mountain Pose (page 27). Keeping your hips level throughout the pose, place the heel and sole of your right foot along your left inner thigh. Press your big toe and inner edge of foot into your inner thigh and firm your thigh against the contact. Move your right knee back so it's in line with both hips. Inhale as you arc your arms out to the sides and over your head to press your palms together. Drop your shoulders back and away from your ears as you continue extending upward.

Hold for 10 breaths. Repeat on the other side.

Sideways Extension
(Parsvottanasana)

■ *parsva* = side; *tan* = to extend ■ (pars-vuh-tan-AHS-anna) ■

GENERAL BENEFITS: Stretches the spine, hamstrings, shoulders, wrists, and hips; strengthens the ankles, legs, and knees

MODIFICATION: If you cannot press your palms together, hold your elbows instead.

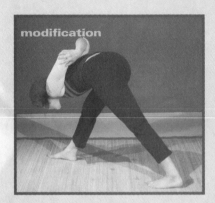

modification

Martial arts application

BENEFITS: Improves balance for all kicks; improves range of motion in linear kicks such as front and axe kicks

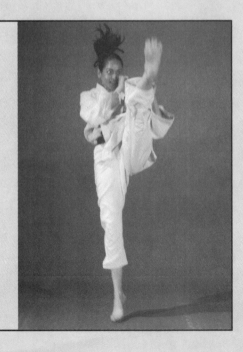

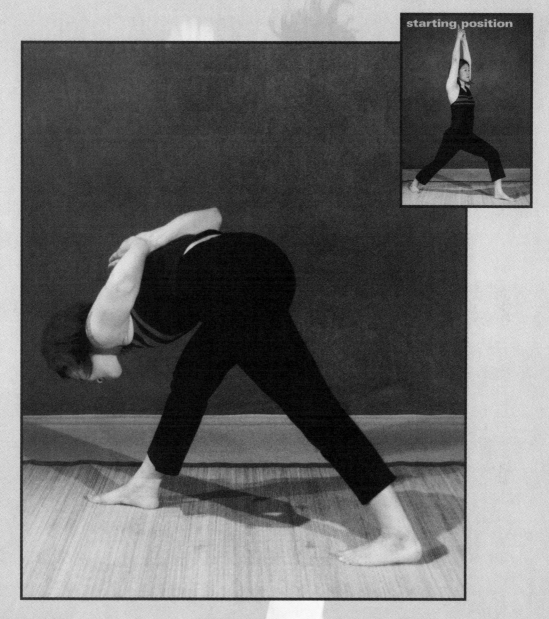

starting position

GETTING INTO POSE: Move from Mountain Pose (page 27) into Warrior I (page 28), right knee bent forward. Press both palms behind your back so that your fingers point to the ceiling. Straighten your front leg, lifting your kneecap toward your hip. Inhale to extend your chest, waist, and hips up. Exhale to fold forward from your hips, bringing chest to thigh and chin to shin. Keep the hips level and continue pressing firmly into both feet.

Hold for 10 breaths. Repeat on the other side.

Half Moon (Ardha Chandrasana)

■ *ardha* = half; *chandra* = glittering, shining (or moon) ■
(ar-dah chan-DRAHS-anna) ■

GENERAL BENEFITS: Improves balance and coordination; strengthens the legs, ankles, thighs, abdominals, and butt; stretches the groin muscles, legs, shoulders, and chest

MODIFICATION: Place your lower hand on a block or book and/or use a wall to support your back and legs.

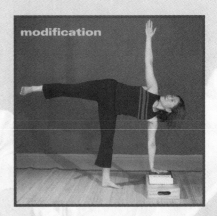

modification

Martial arts application

BENEFITS: Improves balance for all kicks; teaches proper alignment of hips and legs for the side kick; strengthens the muscles of the hip/torso/butt that hold up your side kick and similar kicks such as hook and roundhouse kicks

CHALLENGE: Without compromising your feet/leg/torso positioning (although you can lower your raised leg if it's higher than your hips), bring your lower hand to your sternum and contract your oblique muscles, lifting your torso to place your top arm along your extended leg.

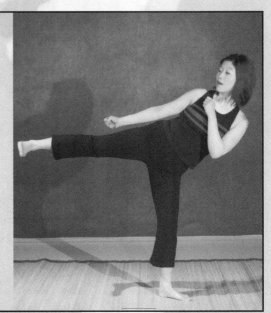

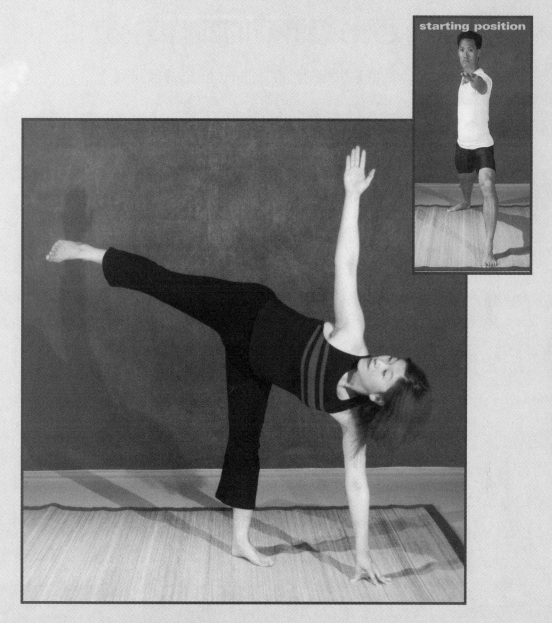

starting position

GETTING INTO POSE: Move from Mountain Pose (page 27) to Warrior II (page 28), left knee bent. Keeping your chest and hips facing forward, exhale and reach your left hand to the floor in front of your left foot as you raise your right leg parallel to the ground or in line with the side of your torso, toes and knee pointing forward. Straighten your left knee. Your arms should form one line from ceiling to floor. Turn your head to gaze softly beyond your top hand.

Hold for 5 breaths. Repeat on the other side.

Warrior III (Virabhadrasana III)

■ Virabhadra = a mighty warrior who was an incarnation of Shiva ■
(veer-ah-bah-DRAHS-anna) ■

GENERAL BENEFITS: Improves balance and coordination; strengthens the ankle, legs, butt, torso; promotes body coordination

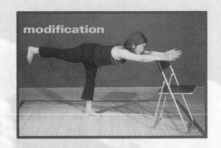
modification

MODIFICATION: Practice this with a chair in front of you so you can lightly touch the top of it for support as you extend both arms and leg.

ADVANCED: Begin in Sideways Extension Pose (page 96) with your hands on either side of your front foot. Raise and extend both your arms and back leg until they are parallel to the ground.

Martial arts application

BENEFITS: Improves balance for all kicks; strengthens the muscles used in back kicks

CHALLENGE: Keeping your torso and arms parallel to the floor, lower your raised leg until your toes touch the floor, then lift it back to parallel. Repeat 4 more times.

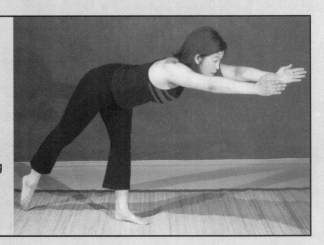

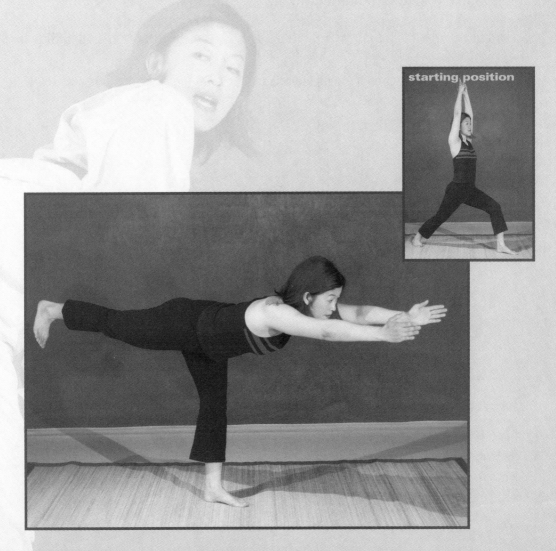

starting position

GETTING INTO POSE: Move from Mountain Pose (page 27) into Warrior I (page 28), left knee bent forward. Exhale and extend your torso over your front leg, bringing your arms, torso, and back leg parallel to the floor. Keeping your hips and back level, reach your fingertips forward and your foot behind you. Gaze softly beyond your extended fingers.

Hold for 5 breaths. Release by inhaling back to Warrior I. Repeat on the other side.

Reverse Triangle
(Parivrtta Trikonasana)

■ *parivrtta* = reverse; *trikona* = three angle ■ (par-ee-vrit-tah trik-cone-AHS-anna) ■

GENERAL BENEFITS: Stretches the hips, spine, and legs; strengthens the legs and ankles; opens the chest; improves balance

Martial arts application

BENEFITS: Improves balance for all kicks; improves spine and hip flexibility for all kicks, including spinning and turning ones

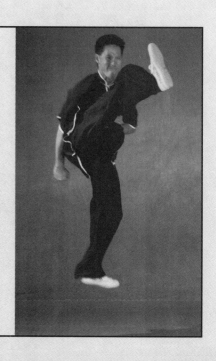

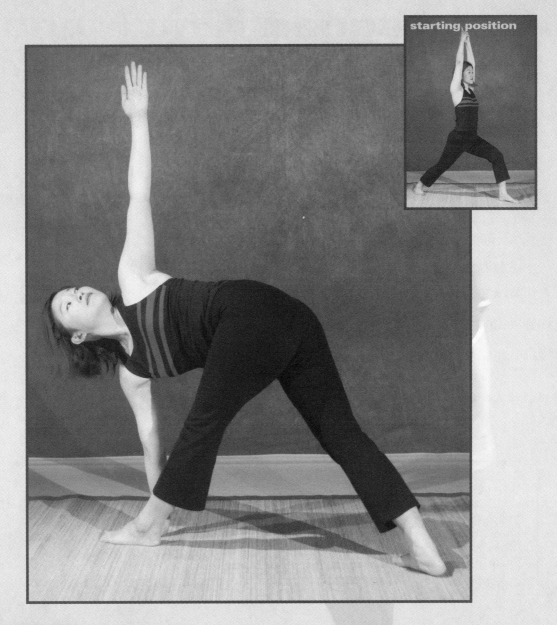

starting position

GETTING INTO POSE: Move from Mountain Pose (page 27) into Warrior I (page 28), left knee bent forward. Straighten your front leg, lifting your kneecap toward your hip. Inhale to extend your chest, waist, and hips up. Exhale to fold forward from your hips and place both hands firmly on the ground on either side of your foot. Keeping your hips aligned, inhale to circle your right arm alongside your body, opening your torso toward the right, until your arm is perpendicular to the floor and palm faces forward. Turn your head to gaze at your top hand.

Hold for 5 breaths. Repeat on the other side.

One-Legged King Pigeon
(Eka Pada Rajakapotasana)

■ *eka* = one; *pada* = leg; *raja* = king; *kapota* = pigeon ■
(aa-KAH pah-DAH rah-JAH-cop-poh-TAHS-anna) ■

Commonly known as Pigeon Pose

Note: This is a "kicks" variation of the full pose, which is actually a backbend in addition to an intense stretch of the hips, quads, and groin muscles.

GENERAL BENEFITS: Stretches the hips, quads, and groin muscles

VARIATION 1: You can also rest your forearms on the floor.

VARIATION 2: Reach behind with your right hand to grasp the foot of your bent right leg, keeping your hips equidistant from the floor.

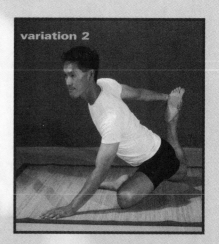
variation 2

Martial arts application

BENEFITS: Releases hip flexors for faster/easier knee lifting; improves hip flexibility for side, roundhouse, hook, and butterfly kicks

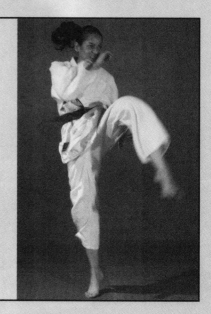

The Martial Artist's Book of Yoga

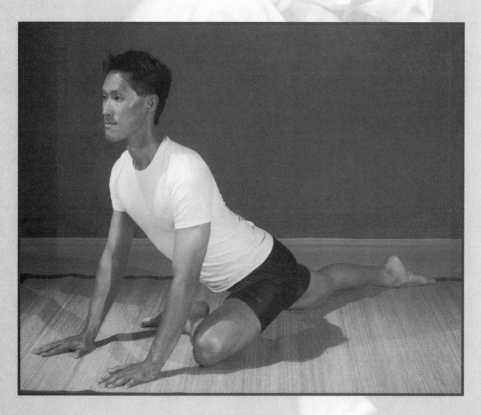

GETTING INTO POSE: Start on your hands and knees, with hands below shoulders and knees below hips. Slide your left knee to your left wrist and angle your foot so that it's by your right knee. Rest your shin on the floor and extend your right leg back, releasing the thigh to the floor. Keep your head aligned with your spine and your hips equidistant from the floor so your pelvis is not leaning to one side.

Hold for 10 breaths. Repeat on the other side.

Seated Angle (Upavishta Konasana)

■ *upavishta* = seated, sitting; *kona* = angle ■ (oo-pah-VEESH-tah cone-AHS-anna) ■

GENERAL BENEFITS: Stretches the legs and groin; strengthens the back

MODIFICATION: If you cannot reach your toes, loop a belt around each foot and gently pull.

VARIATION: Bring your belly, then chest, then head to the floor.

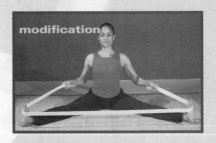

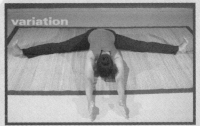

Martial arts application

BENEFITS: Improves range of motion for linear kicks; prevents hunching when kicking by teaching good posture

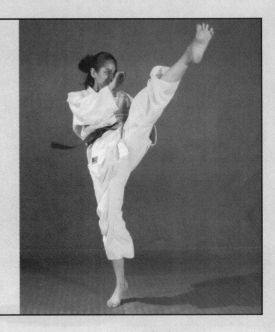

The Martial Artist's Book of Yoga

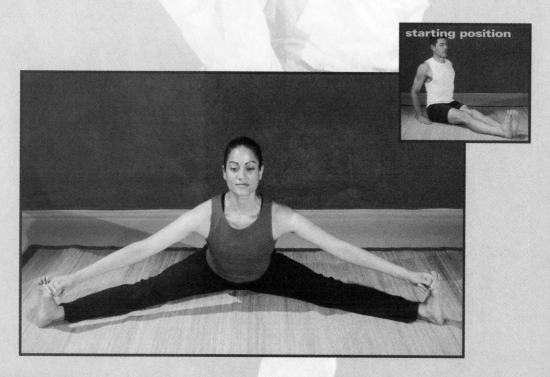

starting position

GETTING INTO POSE: Begin in Staff Pose (page 31). Exhale and simultaneously spread both legs wide apart, with both knees and toes pointing toward the ceiling. Keeping your legs straight and lifting your kneecaps to your hips, inhale and press your hands on the floor behind your hips to extend and open your chest. Exhale to fold forward from your hips and reach your fingers to your toes.

Hold for 10 breaths.

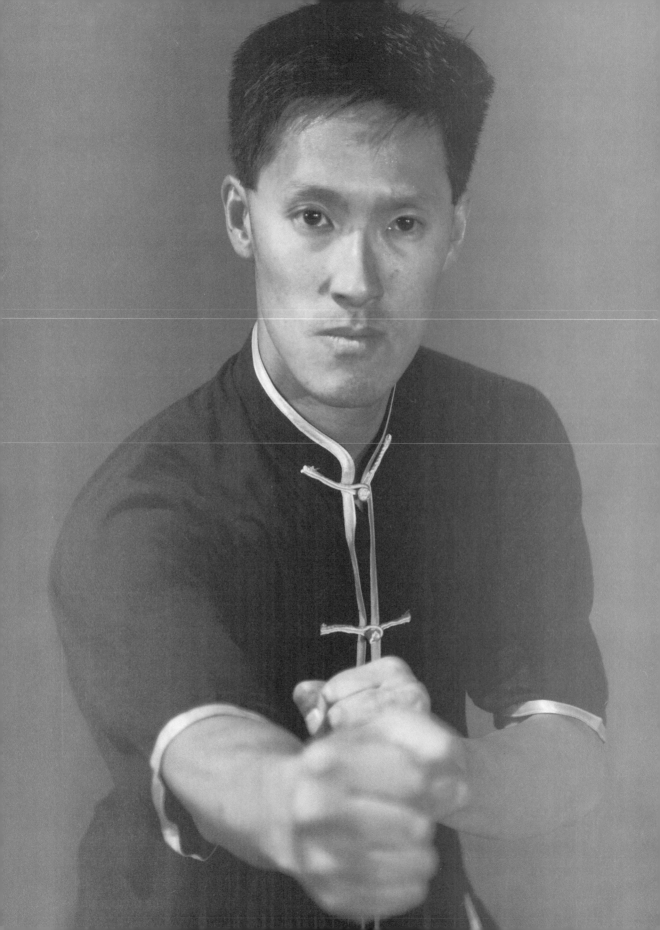

Strikes/Blocks

Using arms and hands to strike or block is perhaps the most common, innate reaction in a close-contact situation. Although hand and elbow strikes may not be as powerful as kicks, they can be very effective and often more accurate than kicks. The arm's range of motion and the hand's ability to change form and striking surface allow for a large variety of techniques: front punch, upper-cut, backfist, rising block, Y block, spearhand, knife hand, palm heel—to name but a few. The degree of impact made by any of these depends not only on hand and arm strength but on the coordination of the entire body and breath.

KEY ANATOMY

Strikes and blocks are delivered using the entire upper body (arms, shoulders, chest, elbows, fingers, hands), with the hips and legs providing significant power.

Essential Elements

BODY AWARENESS/CONTROL While even poorly executed blocks may still prevent maximum damage to your body, inaccurate strikes are basically useless (unless they succeed in distracting your aggressor, enabling you to follow up with another technique) and can actually throw you off balance and/or make you vulnerable to counterattacks. Hitting your target requires hand-eye coordination, but this is just the first step in carrying out an effective technique. Striking and blocking with power also involves timing, the coordination of your legs, hips, back, and shoulders, as well as the last-minute twist of the arm you're using. Part of this power stems from keeping your elbows close to your power source (your hips) and not rotating your shoulders away from the direction of the strike/block. In addition, a relaxed body contributes speed and power by allowing your body to react like a whip.

BODY ALIGNMENT When engaging your arms and hands as weapons or shields, you need to make sure they're as sturdy and unyielding as, say, a stick, a knife, or a suit of armor. Instruments with any degree of pliancy (such as plastic knives) will either snap or give way under pressure. Your arms and hands will fail similarly if they're not aligned properly, which is why it's crucial to create and maintain a strong, straight line from your shoulder or elbow to your striking surface, depending on the technique. A line from your striking surface through your arm, shoulder, back, and legs is often also important for power.

FLEXIBILITY The rate at which you can extend your arm determines the speed of your strike or block. The speed of extension and retraction, combined with the synchronized movements of your hips and legs, determines the power of the strike or block. Flexible shoulders, hips, and spine benefit both functions. Since the

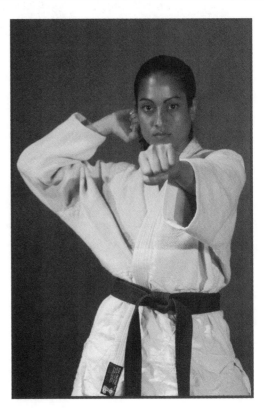

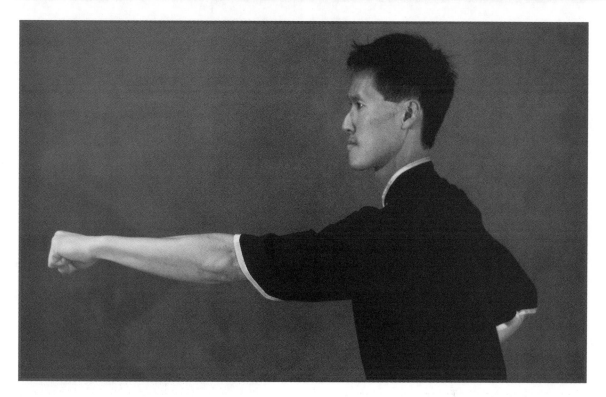

core transfers the power generated by your legs and hips into your upper body, a supple spine contributes greatly to power and speed. Limber shoulders also allow greater range of motion and reach.

BREATH CONTROL Emitting a *kihap/kiai* ("spirit yell") as you strike/block accomplishes more than drawing attention to your movements. Exhaling explosively as you strike/block focuses all your attention on that technique and provides concentrated power by channeling your internal energy outward through your arm/hand. Controlling your breath also improves aerobic capacity and delivery of oxygen to your muscles.

Benefits of Yoga

The Fundamental poses increase the speed and power of your hand techniques by strengthening your stances and improving the alignment and range of motion of your hips, spine, and arms. The poses in this section build on those benefits primarily by working the upper body. They strengthen the arms and wrists to better deliver hand techniques, promote good alignment of the shoulders, and emphasize the connection between elbows and torso. They also reverse the inflexibility that comes from overusing your shoulders and the main culprit of day-to-day tightness for many of us: hunching over a desk or computer for hours at a time.

Poses for Strikes/Blocks

Four-Limbed Staff (*Chaturanga Dandasana*)

Vasishta's Pose (*Vasishtasana*)

Triangle (*Trikonasana*)

Crane (*Bakasana*)

One-Legged Downward-Facing Dog (*Eka Pada Adho Mukha Svanasana*)

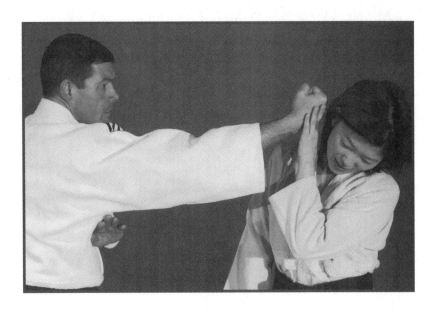

Other Poses

These poses that appear elsewhere in the book also benefit strikes and blocks:

Bow *(page 66)*: stretches the chest and shoulders

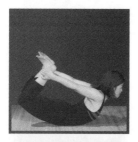

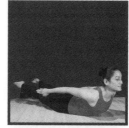

Locust *(page 46)*: strengthens the arms, legs, and back; stretches the chest and shoulders

Cowface *(page 60)*: stretches the upper body and hips

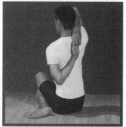

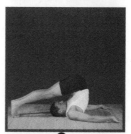

Plow *(page 50)*: stretches the shoulders and spine

Eagle *(page 132)*: improves balance; stretches the hips and shoulders

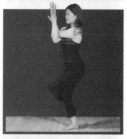

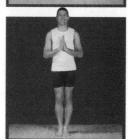

Prayer *(page 78)*: improves wrist flexibility

Sideways Extension *(page 96)*: stretches the shoulders, wrists, and legs

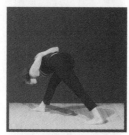

Front Extension *(page 82)*: conditions the arms and wrists

Intense Leg Extension III *(page 80)*: stretches the shoulders and legs

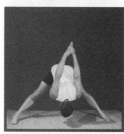

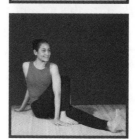

Marichi's Pose III *(page 140)*: stretches the shoulders; promotes spine mobility for better transfer of power

Four-Limbed Staff
(Chaturanga Dandasana)

■ *chatur* = four; *anga* = limb; *danda* = staff ■ (chaht-tour-ANG-ah don-DAHS-anna) ■

GENERAL BENEFITS: Strengthens the arms, wrists, and abs; teaches proper shoulder/head/neck alignment

Martial arts application

BENEFITS: Helps improve power by keeping elbows in; improves wrist flexibility for palm heel strikes

CHALLENGE: Keeping your elbows by your sides, push all the way up until your body is one diagonal line from head to heels (also known as Plank). Perform this lift and lower 5 times.

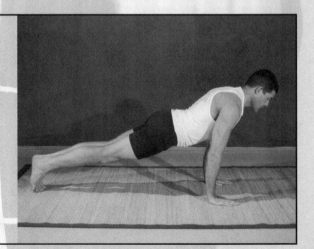

The Martial Artist's Book of Yoga

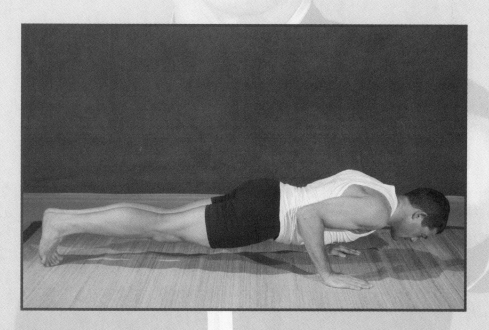

GETTING INTO POSE: Lie face down with your legs extended along the floor. Place your hands beneath your shoulders, fingers spread wide apart, and your elbows by your sides. Tuck your toes under and inhale. Exhale and, continuing to keep your elbows by your sides, push into your hands and toes to raise your entire body just a few inches off the ground. Keep your body in one line and your ears aligned with your shoulders.

Hold for 5 breaths.

Vasishta's Pose (Vasishtasana)

■ Vasishta = name of a sage ■ (vah-sish-TAHS-anna) ■

Commonly known as **Side Plank**

GENERAL BENEFITS: Strengthens the arms, wrists, abs, and legs; stretches the wrists; improves balance

VARIATION: Bend your left knee to your chest and hold the toes with your left hand before straightening your leg to the ceiling.

Martial arts application

BENEFITS: Improves extension of strikes/ blocks; improves wrist flexibility for palm heel strikes

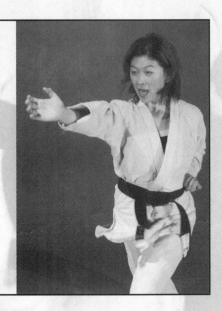

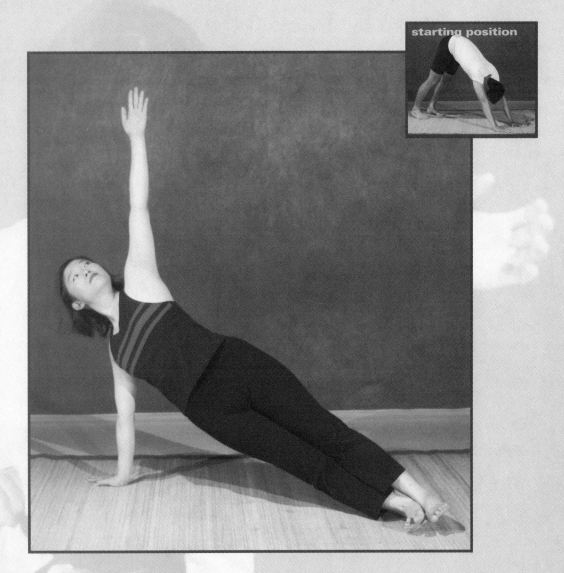

starting position

GETTING INTO POSE: Begin in Downward-Facing Dog Pose (page 30). Lower your pelvis until your body forms a straight line from head to feet (also known as Plank Pose). Inhale and shift your weight into your right hand and right foot. Exhale and reach your left hip toward the ceiling to open your torso to the left. As your body opens, allow your right foot to rotate and rest on its outer edge, keeping your leg long and strong. Stack your left foot on top of your right and extend your left arm toward the ceiling. Turn your head to gaze up at your hand.

Hold for 5 breaths.

Triangle (Trikonasana)

■ *trikona* = three angle ■ (trik-cone-AHS-anna) ■

GENERAL BENEFITS: Stretches the shoulders, chest, spine, hips, groin, hamstrings, and calves; stretches and strengthens the quads, knees, and ankles; improves balance

Martial arts application

BENEFITS: Improves extension of strikes/blocks; increases spine and hip flexibility for better transfer of power

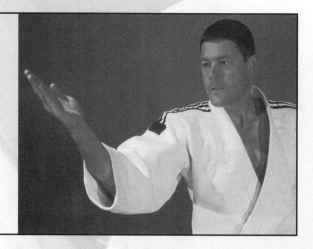

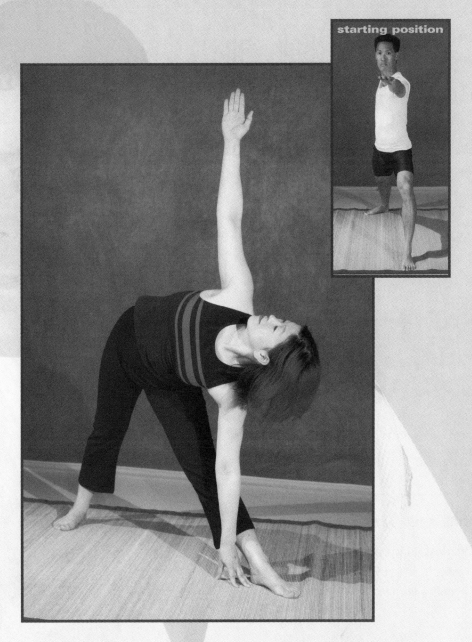

starting position

GETTING INTO POSE: Move from Mountain Pose (page 27) into Warrior II (page 28), left knee bent. Straighten your left leg. Inhale and extend your left arm and your left side over your left leg, placing your hand on your thigh, shin, or floor. Extend your right hand to the ceiling. Turn your head to gaze past your top arm.

Hold for 10 breaths. Repeat on the other side.

Crane (Bakasana)

■ *baka* = crane ■ (bahk-AHS-anna) ■

GENERAL BENEFITS: Strengthens arms, wrists, and abs; stretches the groin muscles; improves balance

Martial arts application

BENEFITS: Improves control, balance, and focus for all strikes; teaches importance of keeping elbows in

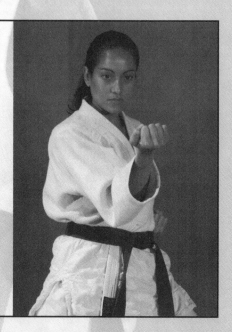

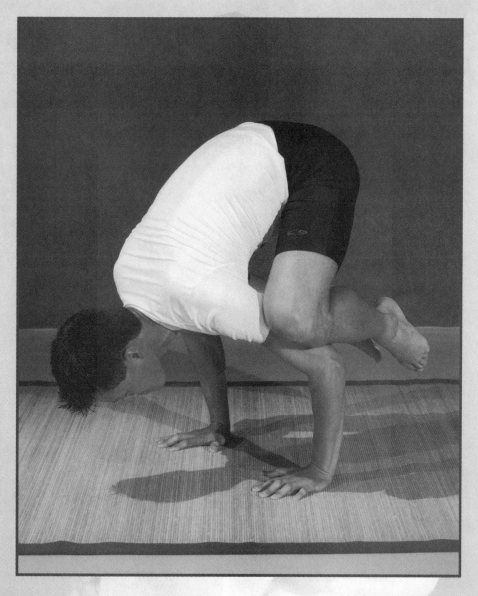

GETTING INTO POSE: Stand with your feet about hip-width apart. Squat down with your upper arms inside your knees. Spread your fingers and place your hands on the floor about 12 inches in front of you. Keeping your heels close to your butt, rise high up onto the balls of your feet and lift your butt to place your shins firmly on your upper arms, with your knees close to your armpits.

Hold for 5 breaths.

One-Legged Downward-Facing Dog
(Eka Pada Adho Mukha Svanasana)

■ *eka* = one; *pada* = leg; *adho* = downward; *mukha* = face; *svana* = dog ■
(aa-KAH pah-DAH AH-doh MOO-kah shvah-NAHS-anna) ■

GENERAL BENEFITS: Strengthens the wrists, arms, shoulders, back, and legs; stretches the hamstrings and calves

Martial arts application

BENEFITS: Improves extension of strikes/
blocks; improves wrist flexibility for palm
heel strikes

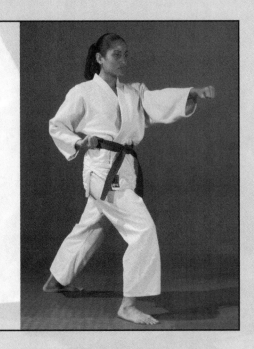

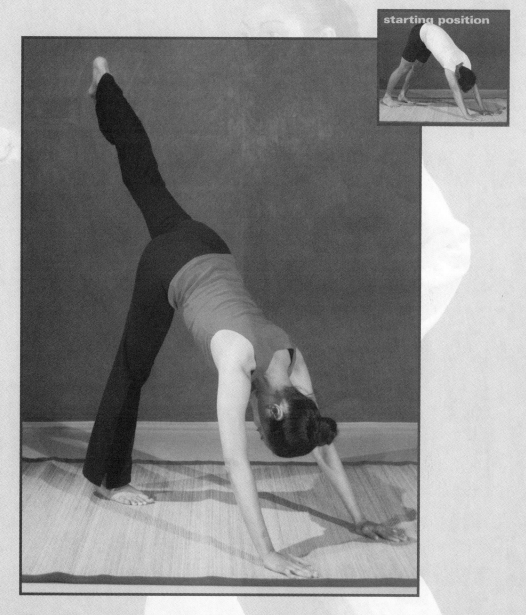

starting position

GETTING INTO POSE: Begin in Downward-Facing Dog Pose (page 30). Keeping your hips level, raise one leg until it is in line with your torso and arms. Lengthen both legs, reaching one foot into the floor and the other heel to the wall behind you. Relax your head between your biceps.

Hold for 5 breaths.

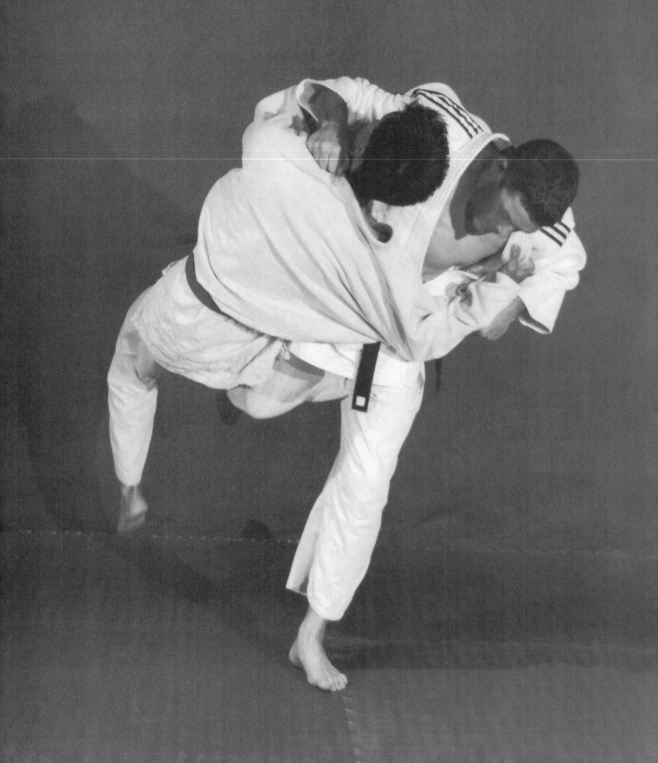

Throwing an opponent involves techniques that maneuver mass using the opponent's momentum and your entire body. Whether you practice them from standing or by engaging in *randori* (the art of moving with your partner and trying to catch her off-balance so you can execute a foot sweep, major outer reap, forward body drop, or some other kind of throw), the goal is the same: to break your partner's balance and take her to the ground. The coordination required by the many exacting movements means that throws demand a lot of practice before they become effective.

KEY ANATOMY

Executing a throw, from the initial balance break to the final takedown, involves the coordination of the whole body.

Essential Elements

BODY AWARENESS/CONTROL Throwing a person requires a complex sequence of moves that involves precise timing and the coordination of many parts of your body. For this reason, you need to be aware of what your body is (and isn't) doing at all times. Did you remember to continue pulling your partner off-balance as you stepped in, squatting below his center of mass? And did you get your hips close enough, and turned just right?

Body awareness is just the beginning of being able to blend all these pieces together into one effective technique. Once you gain control of your body, the synchronization of your movements will improve and the frequency of injury (from incorrectly using your back, shoulders, knees) will decrease. Body control also helps you better regulate the power generated by your movements.

BALANCE Balance plays a critical role in throws. Certainly, the balance of the person to be thrown must be broken, and the person throwing must continue and commit to the momentum (usually by also being off-balance) until the throw is achieved. Since the person throwing generally sets the pivot point of the throw, a good sense of balance is the key to not simply toppling over as you load

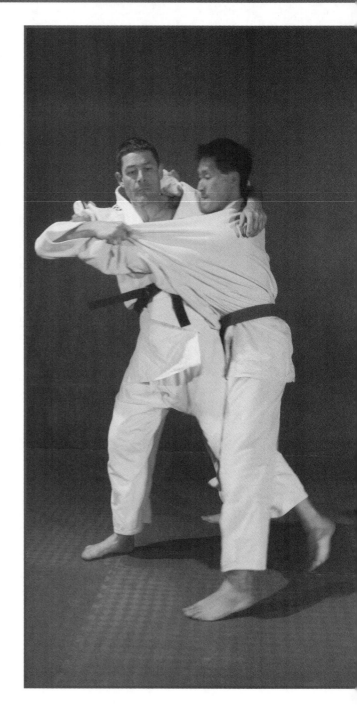

The Martial Artist's Book of Yoga

your partner for a shoulder throw or being swept off your feet when you attempt a major outer reap. Having a good sense of balance also helps you regain your footing much more quickly, whether you've completed a throw or your partner has tried to break your balance in a round of *randori*.

BODY ALIGNMENT To execute a throw, your feet and hips must be placed correctly in relation to your partner. Footwork is crucial, too, but you'll find that if parts of your body aren't in proper anatomical alignment (say, one hip is always ahead of the other or your feet turn out), it takes extra effort to get into position. Good body alignment allows less readjustment of form/body placement. It also assures that the correct muscles are being used for that particular function, resulting in safer and more efficient throws.

FLEXIBILITY Although some lack of flexibility won't limit your throwing as much as it would affect your kicking (not being able to do full splits, for instance, won't prevent you from being an Olympic-grade judoka), a moderate degree of flexibility enables you to move into and execute techniques smoothly and quickly. Since throws utilize the whole body, hav-

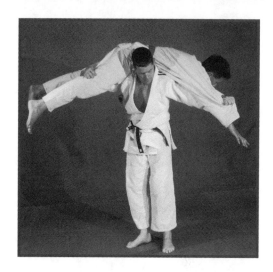

ing a supple spine is important because the core transfers the power of your hips and legs into your upper body; additionally, you'll be less likely to pull something when you inadvertently use your back to throw your partner.

Flexibility in other parts of your body also enhances your ability to throw. Loose hips allow faster footwork, whether to get into position or quickly switch the kind of throw you want to do. Good range of motion in your knees makes it easier to get below or around your partner's center of mass. Flexible shoulders are more resilient to the strain that comes from accidentally leaving your shoulder behind (that is, not keeping your shoulders aligned with the rest of your upper body as you rotate) while throwing.

Benefits of Yoga

The Fundamental poses aid throwing techniques by encouraging proper body alignment, flexibility of the hips, shoulders, and spine, and strengthening the legs. The poses in this section build on these benefits and also improve balance. Several improve the range of motion in your knees by maintaining the muscular balance of your hamstrings and quads, which are often overworked from repeated squatting.

Poses for Throws

Powerful (*Utkatasana*)

Eagle (*Garudasana*)

Reverse Half Moon (*Parivrtta Ardha Chandrasana*)

Cobra (*Bhujangasana*)

Intense Stretch of the West (*Paschimottanasana*)

Marichi's Pose III (*Marichyasana III*)

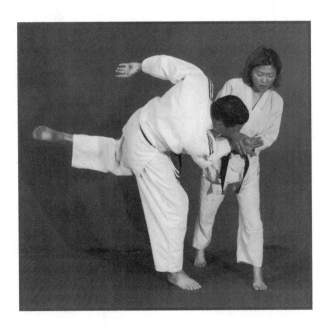

Other Poses

These poses that appear elsewhere in the book also benefit throws:

Bharadvaja's Pose I *(page 44)*: improves spine and hip mobility

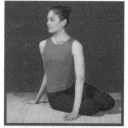

Plow *(page 50)*: stretches the shoulders and spine

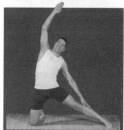

Gate *(page 40)*: stretches the sides of the body and hips

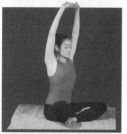

Front Extension *(page 82)*: conditions the upper body for stronger off-balancing pulls

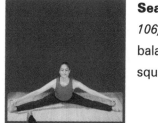

Happy Mountain *(page 84)*: stretches the hips and upper body

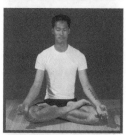

Seated Angle *(page 106)*: restores muscular balance after repeated squatting movements

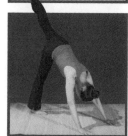

Lotus *(page 86)*: stretches the lower body

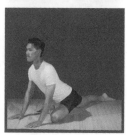

One-Legged Downward-Facing Dog *(page 122)*: strengthens the upper body for stronger off-balancing pulls

One-Legged King Pigeon *(page 104)*: improves hip flexibility; stretches the quads

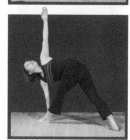

Reverse Triangle *(page 102)*: improves balance for reaping/sweeping throws; improves hip and spine flexibility

Powerful (Utkatasana)

■ *utkata* = powerful ■ (OOT-kah-TAHS-anna) ■

Also known as **Chair Pose**

GENERAL BENEFITS: Strengthens the shoulders, arms, abs, back, knees, quads, and ankles; improves ankle stability

VARIATION: Starting in Intense Stretch Pose (page 29), bend your knees. Keeping your biceps by your ears, reach your arms and torso forward and up.

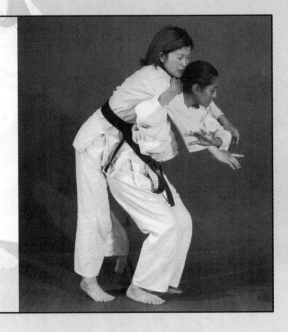

Martial arts application

BENEFITS: Conditions the knees and hips for the squatting movement involved in forward throws

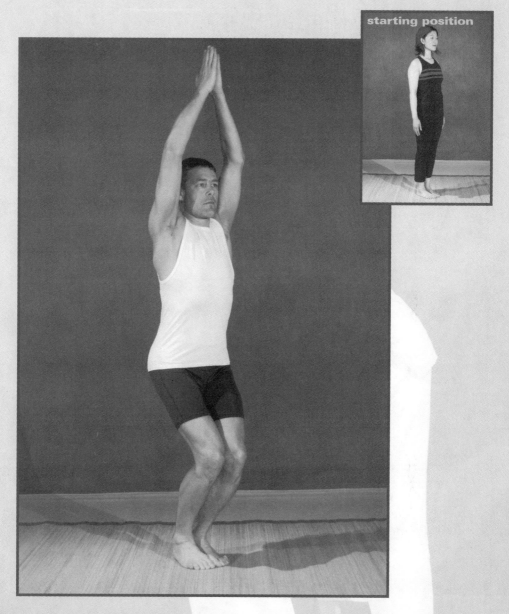

starting position

GETTING INTO POSE: Begin in Mountain Pose (page 27). Inhale and reach your arms above your head, pressing your palms together or interlocking your fingers and pointing your index fingers to the ceiling. Exhale and bend your ankles, knees, and hips, reaching your hips back and down as if to sit. Although your torso will naturally lean forward, keep your back straight and continue reaching upward as your hips reach down.

Hold for 10 breaths.

Eagle (Garudasana)

■ Garuda = the "king of the birds" ■ (gah-rue-DAHS-anna) ■

GENERAL BENEFITS: Strengthens the legs and ankles; stretches the shoulders, arms, wrists, and hips; improves balance and ankle stability

Martial arts application

BENEFITS: Reverses the effect of leaving the shoulder behind; improves balance for reaping/sweeping throws; improves hip flexibility for better transfer of power for all throws

CHALLENGE: Fold forward from your hips until your torso is parallel to the floor. Hold for one breath before returning to standing. Repeat 4 more times.

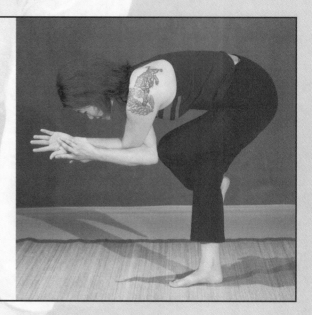

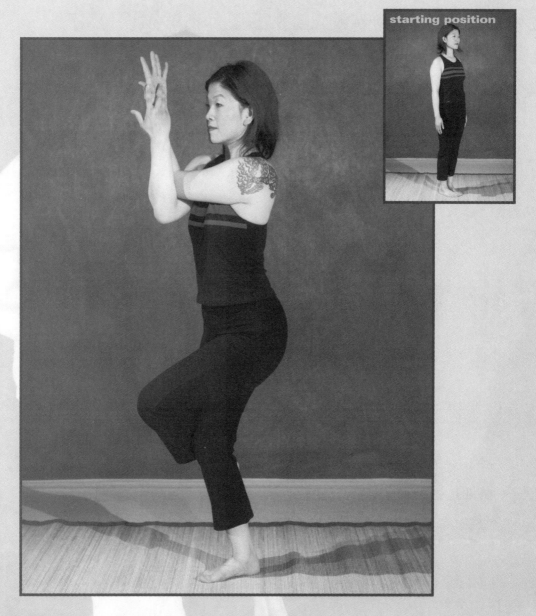

starting position

GETTING INTO POSE: Begin in Mountain Pose (page 27). Place your hands on your hips and bend your knees. Keeping your hips where they are, cross your left knee over your right and tuck your left foot behind your right calf. Draw your left arm across your face and cross your right elbow below it. Turn your hands to place your right fingers on your left palm. Raise your elbows to shoulder height and draw your shoulder blades back and down.

Hold for 10 breaths. Repeat on the other side.

Reverse Half Moon
(Parivrtta Ardha Chandrasana)

■ *parivrtta* = reverse; *ardha* = half; *chandra* = glittering, shining (or moon) ■
(par-ee-vrit-tah ar-dah chan-DRAHS-anna) ■

GENERAL BENEFITS: Stretches the hips, spine, and legs; strengthens legs, ankles; opens the chest; improves balance

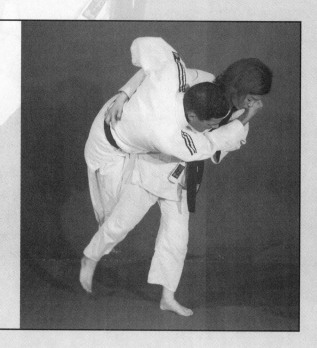

Martial arts application

BENEFITS: Improves balance for reaping/ sweeping throws; improves spine and hip flexibility for better transfer of power for all throws

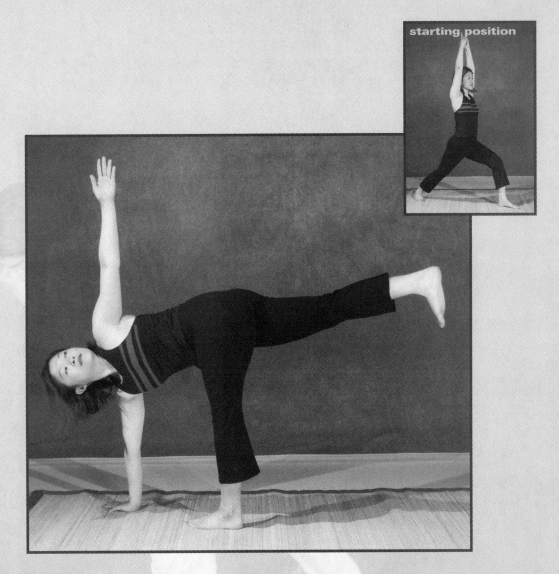

starting position

GETTING INTO POSE: Move from Mountain Pose (page 27) to Warrior I (page 28), left knee bent forward. Fold over your knee to place your hands on either side of your left foot. Move your right hand about 12 inches in front of your foot. Exhale and straighten your knee as you lift your right leg parallel to the floor, knee and toes pointing down. Inhale to circle your left arm alongside your body, opening your torso toward the left, until your arm is perpendicular to the floor and palm faces forward. Gaze up at your top hand.

Hold for 5 breaths. Repeat on the other side.

Cobra (Bhujangasana)

■ *bhujanga* = serpent ■ (boo-jang-GAHS-anna) ■

GENERAL BENEFITS: Strengthens the spine and butt; stretches the chest, shoulders, and abs

Martial arts application

BENEFITS: Reverses the hunched-over posture common among beginners

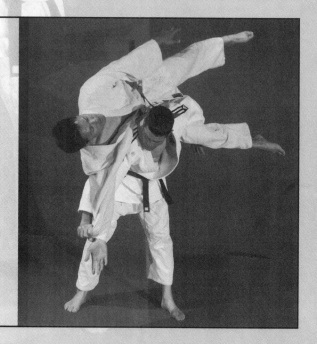

The Martial Artist's Book of Yoga

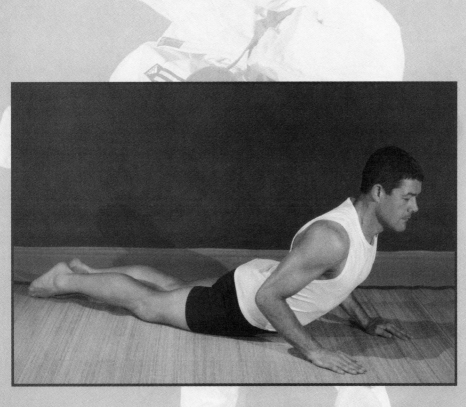

GETTING INTO POSE: Lie face down with your legs extending behind you and palms placed near your waist, forearms vertical to the floor. Keeping your elbows next to your body, press into your hands to lift your chest off the floor. Drop your shoulders away from your ears.

Hold for 5 breaths.

Intense Stretch of the West (Paschimottanasana)

■ *pashima* = west; *uttana* = intense stretch ■ (POSH-ee-moh-tan-AHS-anna) ■

Commonly known as Seated Forward Bend Pose

GENERAL BENEFITS: Stretches the shoulders, spine, and hamstrings

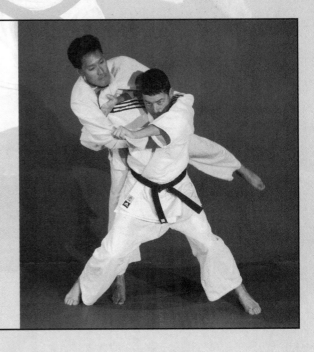

Martial arts application

BENEFITS: Restores muscular balance after repeated squatting movements

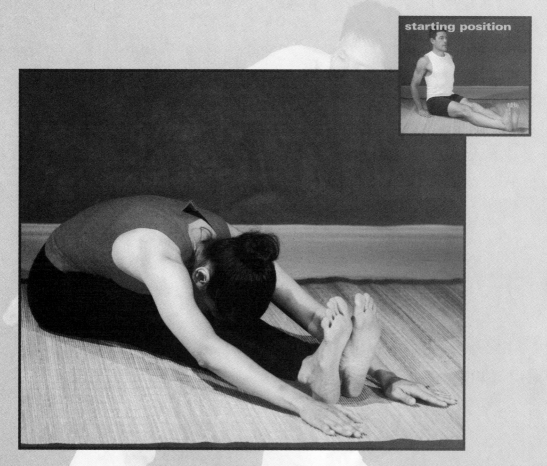

GETTING INTO POSE: Begin in Staff Pose (page 31). Exhale and fold forward from your hips, reaching your chest forward and your hands toward your toes. Hold the sides of your feet or place your hands on the floor, bringing your belly to your thighs and your face to you shins.

Hold for 10 breaths.

Marichi's Pose III
(Marichyasana III)

■ Marichi = name of a sage ■ (mar-ee-chee-AHS-anna) ■

GENERAL BENEFITS: Stretches the shoulders, spine, hips, and outer thighs

VARIATION: As you turn your head to gaze over your right shoulder, move your right hand toward your left hip and slip your left arm through your raised knee to grasp your right hand.

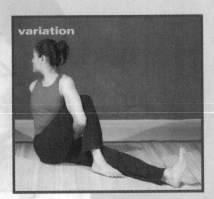

variation

Martial arts application

BENEFITS: Improves spine and hip flexibility for better transfer of power with all throws

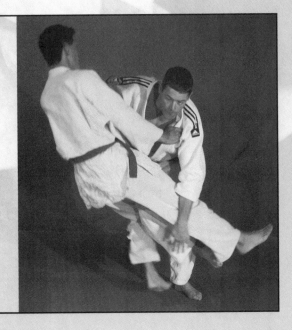

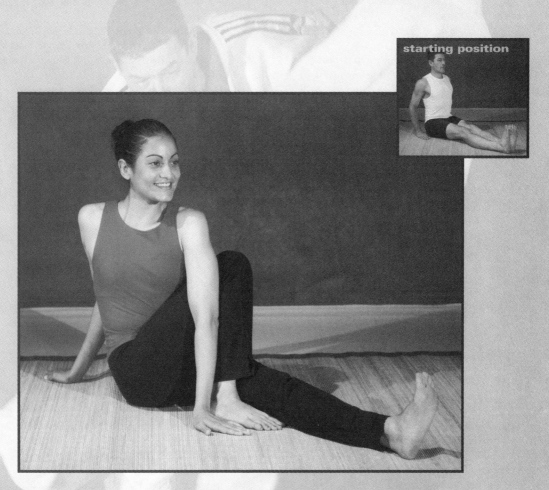

starting position

GETTING INTO POSE: Begin in Staff Pose (page 31). Bend your right leg and, with your foot on the floor, pull your heel in close to your right hip. Exhale and, starting from your tailbone, twist your torso to the right, placing your right hand next to your right hip as your left elbow draws across your body and presses against the outside of your right knee. Gaze over your left shoulder.

Hold for 5 breaths, then gaze over your right shoulder and hold for 5 more breaths. Repeat on the other side.

Index

About the Authors and Photographer

LILY CHOU holds a second-degree black belt in the mixed martial art of yongmudo (formerly known as hapkido) and is an instructor in the Martial Arts Program at the University of California at Berkeley. Her ten years of martial arts training have also included taekwondo; four years of hatha yoga have improved her physical, mental, and spiritual health. As an editor, she has worked on dozens of health and fitness titles for Ulysses Press, including *Yoga for 50+*, *Sexy Yoga*, *Fit in 15*, *Ellie Herman's Pilates Props Workbook*, and *Ultimate Core Ball Workout*. She lives and trains in Berkeley, California.

KATHE ROTHACHER, a kinesiologist, teaches various movement systems and methods, among them Feldenkrais, yoga, Pilates, and dance; she has been practicing yoga for over 30 years. She enjoys the combination of a thriving private practice and her work at the University of California at Berkeley and the Claremont Resort & Spa with her interest of family and personal growth. She lives in Kensington, California, with her husband and children.

ANDY MOGG is a well-known and much-published photographer. Born in England in 1954, he worked as a consultant, then writer and photographer. At 17, he moved from London to Belgium, traveling and working his way through Europe; he settled in the U.S. 20 years ago. He now runs a thriving photography studio in San Francisco. For more information, visit his website at www.dancingimages.com.

Acknowledgments

Many thanks to all at Ulysses Press for making this book a reality. Much admiration to Andy Mogg and his skill in capturing the beauty inherent in yoga and the martial arts. Much appreciation and respect to Dr. Norman Link, whose knowledge and experience have been invaluable in the writing of this book; his unflagging energy and dedication to the martial arts are also an inspiration. Thanks to the models for being a pleasure to work with, both on and off the mat: Jon Bertsch, head judo instructor in the Martial Arts Program at the University of California at Berkeley, is a 25-year martial arts veteran with a 4th *dan* in judo and a 1st *dan* in hapkido; Adriana Espinosa, who has been training for nearly three years, is a 2nd *kub* in yongmudo; Percy Luu, a student of Chinese martial arts for eight years, has trained in disciplines such as wushu, taijiquan, baguazhang, traditional kung fu, and hapkido. Much gratitude to the Martial Arts Program at the University of California at Berkeley (www.ucmap.org) for providing excellent martial arts instruction for nearly four decades.